Key Issues in Childhood and Youth Studies

Key Issues in Childhood and Youth Studies presents an informed and critical commentary on a range of key issues related to children and childhood, from birth to 18 years. Challenging current orthodoxies within the adult world on the nature of childhood, it is an essential text for students of childhood and youth studies, as well as those studying for relevant professional qualifications in social work, teaching and health.

Exploring ideas from the historical development of childhood to the demonizing of youth, the book is divided into five clearly defined parts, each with its own editorial introduction which highlights the key themes. The parts focus on:

- the concept and creation of childhood
- child development
- ideas of risk, protection and childhood
- the politics of childhood
- international perspectives on childhood.

This invaluable textbook provides an overview of childhood and youth studies and encourages students to think about the issues discussed and to develop their own ideas. Each chapter contains student activities, key points boxes, recommended further reading and a reflection exercise.

Derek Kassem is Principal Lecturer/ Deputy Centre Leader in the Centre for Education Studies and Primary Education at Liverpool John Moores University, with responsibility for both Early Childhood Studies and Education Studies.

Lisa Murphy is Principal Lecturer/ Deputy Centre Leader with responsibility for Primary Education within the Centre for Education Studies and Primary Education at Liverpool John Moores University.

Elizabeth Taylor is Senior Lecturer at Liverpool John Moores University.

Key Issues in Childhood and Youth Studies

Edited by Derek Kassem, Lisa Murphy and Elizabeth Taylor

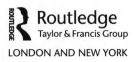

LONDON AND NEW YORK

First published 2010
by Routledge
2 Park Square, Milton Park, Abingdon, Oxon, OX14 4RN

Simultaneously published in the USA and Canada
by Routledge
270 Madison Avenue, New York, NY 10016

Routledge is an imprint of the Taylor & Francis Group, an informa business

Typeset in Garamond by Pindar NZ, Auckland, New Zealand
Printed and bound in Great Britain by TJ International Ltd, Padstow, Cornwall

British Library Cataloguing in Publication Data
A catalogue record for this book is available from the British Library

Library of Congress Cataloging in Publication Data
Key issues in childhood and youth studies: critical issues / edited by Derek
Kassem, Lisa Murphy, and Elizabeth Taylor.
   p. cm.
  Includes bibliographical references and index.
  1 Child development. 2. Children. 3. Child welfare. I. Kassem, Derek. II.
Murphy, Lisa, 1969- III. Taylor, Elizabeth, 1970-
  [DNLM: 1. Adolescent Development. 2. Child Development. 3. Adolescent
Behavior. 4. Child Behavior. 5. Child Welfare. WS 105 K44 2010 2010]
  HQ772.K455 2010
  305.231—dc22   2009021808

ISBN10: 0-415-46888-4 (hbk)
ISBN10: 0-415-46889-2 (pbk)
ISBN10: 0-203-86498-0 (ebk)

ISBN13: 978-0-415-46888-6 (hbk)
ISBN13: 978-0-415-46889-3 (pbk)
ISBN13: 978-0-203-86498-2 (ebk)

Contents

Figures

Tables

Activities

Contributors

John Clarke is the Faculty Learning and Development Manager in the Faculty of Education, Community and Leisure at Liverpool John Moores University.

Diahann Gallard is Senior Lecturer in Educational Psychology and Early Years at Liverpool John Moores University.

Diane Grant is Reader in Community and Social Studies at Liverpool John Moores University.

John Harrison is Senior Lecturer in Childhood Studies at Liverpool John Moores University.

Derek Kassem is Principal Lecturer and Deputy Centre Leader at the Centre for Education Studies and Primary Education at Liverpool John Moores University.

Lynne Kendall is Senior Lecturer in Education Studies and Special Needs at Liverpool John Moores University.

Andrew Kennedy is Senior Lecturer in Early Childhood Studies at Liverpool John Moores University.

Heather Montgomery is Senior Lecturer in Childhood and Youth Studies at the Centre for Childhood, Development and Learning at the Open University.

Lisa Murphy is Principal Lecturer and Deputy Centre Leader at the Centre for Education Studies and Primary Education at Liverpool John Moores University.

Shirley J. Pressler is Senior Lecturer in Psychology at the University of Huddersfield.

Samantha Punch is Senior Lecturer in Sociology at the University of Stirling.

Samir Qouta is Head of the Research Department of the Gaza Community Mental Health Project.

John Robinson is an Educational Consultant at the Centre for Urban Education at Manchester Metropolitan University.

Gabriella Torstensson is Senior Lecturer in Early Years and Education Studies at Liverpool John Moores University.

Terry Wrigley is Senior Lecturer in Education at the University of Edinburgh.

Acknowledgements

The editors would like to thank Jackie, Clara, Euan, Robin, Eve, Will and Dave for all their support without which we would not have been able to produce this book.

We would also like to say a big thank you to Grace McInnes and Khanam Virjee, our editor and editorial assistant at Routledge, for all their help, assistance and, above all, understanding over the last year.

Part 1

Creating childhood

I know a lot about children – I used to be one.

— Spike Milligan

As the comment from Milligan above illustrates, in discussions about childhood and children all of us feel able to contribute because it is perhaps one of the few areas in life of which we all have had first-hand experience. No matter what the nature of our childhood, we have all been children, so we have all visited that ephemeral and elusive Neverland – whether as a lost boy or girl or as a fairy prince or princess. Due to this factor, all discussions about childhood and children, even academic debate purporting to rest upon empirical and objective data and research evidence, are bound to be subjective in nature to some degree.

As Murphy, *et al.* (2009: 131) point out, childhood is a difficult concept to define as it is socio-historically and culturally constructed. Therefore, not only will people from different societies and eras have very diverse understandings of what constitutes childhood, but the role of children within society and the obligations of society to children will be very varied.

This book sets out to explore, debate and analyse issues and factors which define and affect perceptions of childhood and the lives of children on an individual, societal and international basis. Within this part we will discuss the origins and construction of the concept of childhood and the child, and childhood identity, both historically and within contemporary society.

The first chapter by Clarke focuses on the debate concerning the emergence of the concept of childhood as played out in the works of social historians such as Ariès (1962) and Pollock (1983). Clarke outlines the *sentiments* approach taken by Ariès and his followers who assert that a change in feelings, and hence valuation, of the child from the seventeenth century onwards, driven to a large extent by expansion of education, led eventually to the child-centred family unit and society of the twentieth century. In other words, childhood is a construct dependent on socio-historical, political and economic factors, which only came into being from the seventeenth century onwards. After acknowledging the numerous criticisms of this approach, such as dependence on generalized and inaccurate sources, for example, paintings and religious tracts, Clarke suggests that, as the conceptualization of childhood in the late twentieth century is related to the destiny of the nation as a whole, it is indeed a social construct.

Pressler's chapter explores three major images or models of childhood and the child which have evolved historically and are still prevalent in contemporary Western society.

She suggests that these images – the angelic, the demonic and the small person models – are constructed by three discourses about childhood and children: the Romantic, the Puritan and the Rights-based discourses respectively. Pressler suggests that the first two models, in alignment with traditional developmental psychology, construct problematized and negative images of the child as dependent, morally immature and in need – as in a process of *becoming* rather than as a *being*. She concludes that in order to construct more positive images of childhood we must move towards more Rights-based discourses of childhood and contemporary developmental psychology which construct children as a people with a voice and with participatory rights in society (see also Chapter 4.3, this volume).

Kassem's chapter focuses on an increasingly important group of children who are often ignored and almost invisible to the rest of society – children of mixed race or dual heritage. The chapter explores how society and those institutions directly responsible for children, such as the school system, respond to dual-heritage children and how these societal responses impact on the individuals who comprise this group, specifically in terms of how these children construct their identities. The discussion points out that, while this group is comprised of children from a large number of cultures and of ethnic group inter-mixing, it is frequently treated as homogenous rather than heterogeneous. The consequences of this are that when moves are made to cater for dual-heritage children, many individuals within this group are overlooked and marginalized.

Society's inability, or indisposition, to meet the individual needs of children of dual-heritage can have a devastating impact on the way these children construct their identities and on how they view society and their place in it. As dual-heritage ethnicity is the fastest-growing population group in the UK at present, Kassem points out that it is vital that the needs of children within this group are meet.

References

Ariès, P. (1962) *Centuries of Childhood*, Harmondsworth: Penguin Books.

Murphy, L., Mufti, E. and Kassem, D. (2009) *Education Studies: An Introduction*, Maidenhead, Berks: Open University Press.

Pollock, L. H. (1983) *Forgotten Children: Parent–Child Relations from 1500 to 1900*, Cambridge: Cambridge University Press.

1.1 The origins of childhood
In the beginning …

John Clarke

Introduction

The experiences of children, their lives and ideas have not played a major part in traditional approaches to history. Historians concerned with great events and great men and women have relegated children to a minor role, except when their fates affected larger concerns, such as the fifteenth century murder of the princes in the tower.

Alternatively, popular historians have constructed *stories* about the early experiences of usually great men which were seen as prefiguring their later greatness. Stories such as James Watt watching his mother's kettle boiling and imagining the operation of the steam engine or George Washington's honesty when accused by his father of chopping down a cherry tree were more to do with establishing aspects of the adult's later character than they were about describing the nature of childhood at the time concerned. Mostly historians ignored childhood in favour of the activities of adults and, as with the experience of women, or the poor they could be accurately described as *hidden from history* (Rowbotham 1977). The movement to develop and extend the study of childhood can be seen as an aspect of the effort by some historians to recover the ordinary lives of the less powerful elements of society from what Thompson describes as the 'enormous condescension of posterity' (1963: 12).

In recent years, however, questions about childhood and its meaning have come to concern a number of historians, most obviously in the debate about whether or not our idea of childhood is, in fact, just something which has been constructed in recent centuries – *an artefact of modernity*. It has been claimed by some theorists and researchers that until the modern period the current idea of childhood simply did not exist. This approach claims that what we now think of as childhood would not have made sense to our ancestors.

It is argued that between about the turn of the seventeenth century and the 1900s, the idea of childhood was invented, and came to be seen as a natural and universally recognized phase of life. This view is most often attributed to the French author, Philippe Ariès, whose book *L'Enfant et la Vie Familiale sous l'Ancien Régime*, translated into English as *Centuries of Childhood*, first published in the 1960s, has been a key element in discussions within the history of childhood ever since. Much of this debate has been highly critical and has involved historians identifying evidence to show that Ariès and his co-thinkers were wrong about the historical facts. However, it is clear that this debate has focused people's attention on what was previously a seriously neglected area of history and has played a major role in the development of the history of childhood as a serious specialism.

Philippe Ariès: childhood as a modern invention

Ariès is associated with a school of history which attempted to shift attention from the kind of traditional history described above, which concentrated on the actions of rulers, warriors, inventors and politicians, onto different aspects of everyday life such as diet, family life or popular customs and practices. This perspective starts out from a view of history which attempts to create an understanding of how people from every part of society made sense of their own lives. This involved examining the question of how ideas and feelings, what the French call *sentiments*, change over time.

Ariès puts forward the idea that the modern world has a view of how people develop from birth to adulthood which is uniquely its own. To simplify, in Ariès' view it could be said that before modernity the key age in development was seven as it was at this point that a person moved out of the family and its protection into a broader social world where they acted as if they were simply smaller versions of the adults around them. In a modern society, however, the age of seven was only a phase in a gradual move from infancy to childhood. Childhood itself was a special state of transition, neither infant nor adult, around which the whole structure of the family had come to operate. Modern society was typically constructed around a separate isolated family unit which was seen as existing primarily to meet the needs of the child. As this idea of the child-centred family is very familiar to us today, it is not easy to accept that it is a recent invention. However, Ariès argued that it is only the changes brought about by societies like Britain, France and the US modernizing their social structure, particularly the development of compulsory schooling, prescribed and provided by the state, which brings about the phase we call childhood.

Without the development of schooling and its consequences in extending the time children depend on their families, this idea of childhood would not have come into existence. Indeed, before modern society was created, it is not clear that there was such an idea at all. In his most extreme and controversial claim, Ariès states: 'in medieval society the idea of childhood did not exist' (1960: 125).

Ariès based his argument on a number of sources of evidence, such as medieval writings on age and development, the portrayal of children and childhood in medieval art, ideas of how children should dress, as well as considering their games and pastimes. Most significantly of all, he studied the way moralists and others wrote about the idea of childhood innocence. This evidence led Ariès to develop his claim about the absence of the idea of childhood in medieval society. For example, his study of medieval art, particularly painting, suggested that in early medieval works children tended to be portrayed as if they were simply scaled down versions of adults. Painting in Europe in the Middle Ages was overwhelmingly dominated by Christian themes. The most common portrayal of a child in medieval European art was the picture of the infant Jesus in all the many paintings of the Madonna and Child. Ariès argues that these portrayals show Jesus as a small version of an adult – faces often have 'older' features and the body shapes are long, muscular and developed. It seems sometimes that it is only the size of the body relative to the surrounding grown-ups which shows that this is a child or a baby. Ariès makes the very strong claim that 'medieval art until the twelfth century did not know childhood or did not attempt to portray it' (ibid.: 31).

Activity 1.1.1: Depictions of children in paintings

By visiting a local gallery or looking at a collection of paintings in books or on the web, see if you can identify examples of where children are depicted.

- Can you pick out examples of children who are presented as small-scale adults?
- How do children differ from adults in their clothes or the way they present themselves?

This view is supported, states Ariès, if we consider children's clothing in the Middle Ages. This was generally made up of outfits which were simply smaller versions of what was fashionable for adults. Babies and infants did have different clothing – they wore baby clothes which were no different for boys and girls – but at about the age of seven both boys and girls moved on to smaller versions of the appropriate adult clothing.

The most controversial aspect of Ariès view relates to the idea that medieval approaches to childhood involved a less intense or attached attitude to children on the part of their parents. It is suggested that parents, particularly fathers, were not so emotionally attached to their children and were consequently less affected by the impact of their children's illness or death.

Ariès' account of the development of ideas of childhood suggests that what we now see as childhood developed from the seventeenth century onwards. This can be seen in painting, for example, by the appearance of works which represent the ordinary everyday lives of children from different walks of life. Ariès describes this as 'a very important point in the history of feelings' (ibid.: 352). The changes in art reflect changes in the way children and childhood are seen.

This shift in attitude is seen by Ariès as an alteration in *sentiment* and takes two forms. The first is that children come to be seen as having a more central role in their families: 'parents begin to recognize pleasure from watching children's antics and "coddling" them' (ibid.: 127). The second change is that writers on morality relationships and conduct come to see children as fragile and in need of protection and guidance. Here Ariès is suggesting that such views had not been common before 1600. Their development in the seventeenth century lays the foundation for modern views of what childhood is.

The main force driving this development, according to Ariès, is the development of formal schooling. This was provided initially for the male children of the aristocracy, but increasingly, as the modern period develops, schooling comes to be seen as desirable or required for all children, whatever their gender or social origins. The significance of schooling for Ariès is that it creates a kind of period of transition or quarantine, not at work and outside the family, for children between infancy and adult life. The gradual extension and intensification of schooling over the period between 1600 and the present day is the basis for defining a new idea of childhood.

It is important, before moving on from the work of Ariès, to remember that he is writing about ideas of childhood, not children themselves. His work is not based on studies of actual children's experiences. He does not draw on first- or second-hand evidence about how children lived or how they were treated. Instead, he discusses ideas of constructs: how people thought about childhood and what the significance of that was for the broader social world. His work played a key role in generating new ideas about children in history. One reason for this was the fact that his ideas were in line with a broader movement of thought about families and family life which came to see recent history as a movement from a time when kinship and close personal relationships were concerned with practical needs and economic necessity, where emotional ties were secondary or unimportant, to a time where the ideal model of the family is of a haven which meets its members needs for love, affection and emotional support. An extreme example of this is in the work of de Mause (1995) who portrays the history of childhood as a progression from classical times, where children were frequently killed or abandoned, through medieval indifference, where wet-nursing and the farming out of children were common, to the present-day emphasis on caring. He states that:

> The history of childhood is a nightmare from which we have only recently begun to awaken. The further back in history one goes, the lower the level of child care, and the more likely children are to be killed, abandoned, beaten, terrorized, and sexually abused.
>
> (1995: 1)

Shorter summarizes this general viewpoint in his claim that 'good mothering is an invention of modernization' (1976: 170). He argues that in traditional societies it was always likely that infants under the age of two would be treated with emotional indifference because the high possibility of infant mortality made parents reluctant to invest emotionally in a life which might very well be quickly snatched away. By contrast, in the twentieth century the welfare of the small child has been given a dominant status in public discourse and this reflects smaller family size, greater prosperity and lower rates of infant death.

Stone (1977), using evidence from the seventeenth century, attempts to show that relations within the family were generally remote and emotionally detached. He points out that the Puritans held an extremely negative view of the child as a sinful being whose will had to be broken by strict discipline, punishment and by denial of pleasure. He suggests that only with the growth of the middle classes, and the stress on individualism, which came with industrialization, did a child-centred view emerge, gradually filtering down from the middle class to the rest of society.

While these historians differ from Ariès in terms of exactly when ideas and practices changed, they share with him a key perspective: what Anderson (1995) calls the *sentiments* approach. What they all agree on is the view that the most important change modernity produced was a shift in patterns of feeling, that is, in the way people understood and valued children. This resulted in an alteration in the emotional meaning and significance of children. The alteration in feelings, from indifference or neutrality to high valuation, eventually resulted in the twentieth-century family, which is built around supportive relationships and seen as child-centred. All the writers would argue that the modern family is focused *emotionally* on the welfare of the child in ways that would have seemed unintelligible to people from earlier times.

Problems with the Ariès approach: how much has childhood changed?

As we have seen, many writers have accepted Ariès' broad approach. His ideas corresponded to a general movement within social history and the sociology of the family, which stressed the idea of a broad march of progress towards the emotionally supportive family unit. However, his work also attracted a wide range of critiques. At the heart of these critiques is an argument that Ariès exaggerates the discontinuities between childhood in the past and in the present. In particular, critics have argued against his assertion that childhood is an invention of modernity and did not exist in the Middle Ages.

Pollock (1983) criticizes Ariès and his followers for their research methods and for the way they use evidence to construct their models of thinking and feeling. She believes that it is important to study *actual* parent–child relationships as they existed in history rather than describe generalized ideas about '*sentiments*'.

Of course real data about childhood in the past is very hard to obtain and always likely to be partial. However, there are sources and they frequently present a different picture from the one offered by Ariès and his followers. Pollock's evidence comes from diaries, autobiographies and other first-hand accounts, which she examined for the period 1500 to 1700. If we scrutinize this data, Pollock argues, the strongest impression is that there is a kind of continuity. Families and childhood did not undergo a sudden or dramatic change. For instance, to show that there was no pattern of indifference or lack of feeling, she quotes numerous examples of grief at infant death, from mothers and fathers, from throughout the period. She also demonstrates that, while there were examples of brutal or harsh treatment of children, there is no evidence that these were routine or normal and they are often quoted in the sources so as to condemn them. Generally, Pollock is sceptical of the value of research, which, like Ariès' book, draws on secondary sources where writers discuss ideas about childhood, rather than the experience of children themselves. She suggests that it is a mistake to base our image of what childhood was like on the texts of advice books, sermons and other documents removed from actual experience. It is as if we could tell what real behaviour in a school was like merely by reading the school rules and the head teacher's speech on prize day. Pollock (1983) recommends that it is of more value to study how people actually lived, and what it was actually like to be a child. When we do this, it indicates that there is much more similarity between families of the past and those of the present day than Ariès and his colleagues would assert.

There is an important point here to note: because the people who kept diaries and recorded their feelings and attitudes in autobiographies, poems, or novels were likely to be better educated, and more affluent, using such sources may give us a biased picture of childhood in past times. Indeed, it is difficult to find sources based on the lives of the poor and the itinerant urban artisan or the rural peasant.

There have been a number of strong critiques of Ariès' specific claims about the Middle Ages. Shahar (1992) argues directly that Ariès is wrong and that there was indeed a concept of childhood in medieval society. She argues that 'a concept of childhood existed' and 'that scholarly acknowledgement of the existence of different stages of childhood was not merely theoretical and that parents invested both material and emotional resources in their offspring' (ibid.: 1).

It is important to stress that Ariès did not try to suggest that there was no such thing as affection for children in the Middle Ages. People having no clear concept of childhood is different from people being indifferent to their children. However, what Ariès does claim is that there was a much clearer sense that from about seven years old people moved out of being infants contained within the family into the broader world where they took their place alongside other adults albeit as young men or young women. What distinguishes modern society is the separation of a distinct childhood sphere between infancy and adulthood, a distinct world of childhood with its own clothes, games and entertainments.

In response to Ariès' use of pictorial and artistic evidence, many critics have pointed out that there were in fact numerous medieval pictures showing the naturalistic portrayal of childhood. What is more, those who painted were not setting out generally to represent the world as it really was – indeed, excessive realism was often frowned upon by religious authorities. Instead they set out to depict the spiritual truth of the scene they depicted. Jesus was shown as older-looking than his age and as larger than might be expected because of his significance as the human Son of God. Spiritually, he was seen as superior to all the adults around him and this was reflected in the painting. In the same way, the spread of naturalistic images of Jesus later in history, such as Raphael's chubby little baby, reflects the fact that religious views were changing to stress more forcefully the *humanity* of Jesus. It was theology which determined the treatment of Jesus and angels, not sentiments about childhood. As for differences in clothing, Elton makes a realistic point about the problems of relying on paintings as a source: 'In everyday life children were indeed dressed differently to adults; they were just put in adult clothes to have their portraits painted' (Elton cited in Evans 1997: 63).

Activity 1.1.2: A Jacobean father's grief

Read this poem by the poet and playwright Ben Jonson (1572–1637) written after the death of his oldest son in 1616.

On My First Son
Farewell, thou child of my right hand, and joy;
My sin was too much hope of thee, lov'd boy.
Seven years thou wert lent to me, and I thee pay.
Exacted by the fate, on the just day.
Oh, could I lose all father now! For why
Will man lament the state he should envy?
To have so soon 'scaped world's and flesh's rage
And, if no other misery, yet age?
Rest in soft peace, and asked, say here doth lie
Ben Jonson his best piece of poetry;
For whose sake, henceforth, all his vows be such
As what he loves may never like too much.
                  (http://www.cwrl.utexas.edu/~bump/E316K/11/11/MYSON.HTML)

- Does it support the idea that parents, especially fathers, were detached and indifferent in the face of child death?
- What does it suggest about attitudes to death and their links with religious faith?

The middle-class family: an ideology of child-centredness

Although there are many substantial criticisms to be made of the approach of Ariès and his co-thinkers, there has emerged a general agreement that something about the role of children in families and in the broader society changed between the seventeenth century and the present day. It is possible to describe what happened as the emergence and then the spread of a *middle-class model* or *ideology of the family*. This is a model of family life and the importance of childhood which is associated with the newly emerging commercial classes in Western Europe and is based on the idea of the self-contained family led by a strong father with a central focus on the upbringing of children. Children are seen as the central part of the family's purpose. Families are primarily mechanisms for the proper upbringing of children and their key function is education. In some cases this version of the family was derived from religious faith.

The Puritan family in England or the American colonies was seen as an institution based on ensuring the salvation of family members by proper education in the rules of good behaviour and the importance of faith (Cox 1996). Children were seen as inherently sinful and in need of guidance. At the extreme they were compared to wild animals whose spirit needed to be broken, often by beatings, in order that they might develop humility and obedience, which would lead them to be good Christians (Ozment 1983). Not all families followed this extreme model, even in Protestant communities. Both Pollock and Cox suggest that once again the generalized accounts of writers who advised on child rearing, and the use of extreme examples as if they were typical, have distorted our view of Puritan families (Cox 1996; Pollock 1983). Indeed, Schama (1987: 495) describes seventeenth-century Protestant Holland as a society 'besotted with the children', where the idea of children and their pastimes played a major part in family life and in art.

What these seventeenth-century models of the family share though is a focus on the child and the importance of education. This emphasis was widespread among the new middle classes and was provided with powerful intellectual support in the eighteenth century by the Enlightenment view that children were *naturally innocent* and needed to be directed by appropriate care and education to become good citizens. This view is best expressed in Rousseau's classic book *Emile* (1762), which sets out a plan for the education of a boy to allow natural curiosity and virtue to flower. This benign child-centredness became popular and was associated with the growth of Romanticism, which saw children as close to nature and in some sense uncorrupted and pure. A fashion developed for child portraits by artists such as Reynolds which stressed innocence and cuteness (Porter 1990: 247).

However, this view was at first largely confined to the enlightened aristocracy and the new middle classes. For the great mass of the population of Western European countries like Britain and France, children's lives were characterized by poverty, hard labour and exploitation. At the end of the eighteenth century in London, for example, 'Huge numbers of children survived on the streets by prostitution, begging boot blacking, mudlarking (scavenging on the Thames mud) and pick pocketing ...' (Pugh 2007: 23). Nationally, child mortality was as high as one in three up to the age of two and of those who survived, one in two died before they were 15. In the workhouses the death rate was over 90 per cent. In this context the choices for parents, especially single mothers who were seen as disgraced and immoral, were bleak and this caused an alarming increase in the number of foundlings, that is, babies left abandoned in churches or hospitals. This situation led to the setting up of foundling hospitals such as that established by Thomas Coram, based on private philanthropy and rooted in the emergent idea of the child as an innocent in need of protection (Pugh 2007).

What can be seen here is the development of a contradiction which was to dominate writing and thinking about childhood through the nineteenth century and into the twentieth. There was a clash between a Romantic idealized view of childhood rooted in eighteenth-century Enlightenment and the brutal reality of most children's lives. In *Oliver Twist* (Dickens 1837) for example, the simplicity and naivety of Oliver is contrasted with the adult corrupt lives of the Artful Dodger and Fagin's gang. Similarly, in Kingsley's *Water Babies* (1863) the chimney boys are shown to be really innocent babies. This view of childhood purity, which itself contrasted with the persistent Puritan view of children's inherently sinful nature, paralleled the nineteenth-century concern to save children from labour and exploitation.

Childhood in the nineteenth century: children without childhood

The growth of industrial production in factories, mines and shipyards, and the accompanying movements of population and growth of towns and cities, led to an intensification of the wretchedness of many children's lives. In pre-industrial, rurally based societies children had suffered poverty and hardship and were key elements of the agricultural or craft workforce. However, the emergence of the industrial factory system led to the growth of the idea of going out to work. This is a concept we now take for granted but the importance of this change during the Industrial Revolution was the clear separation of the workplace from the home and family. This meant that those who worked in the factories and mines travelled to and from their place of work, often enduring as much as a 14-hour day between these travelling times.

These changes were especially significant for children. Child labour was not just an accidental side effect of the process of industrialization. Employers commonly preferred child workers to adults because they were flexible, easy to manage and most significantly, inexpensive. Incomes were such that child labour was not an optional extra for most families: they needed what the children earned in order to survive.

The exploitation of children in the factory system provided a clear contrast to the newly emerging idealization of childhood, which was developed by Romantic poets like Wordsworth and Blake. Heywood (2001) argues that Wordsworth's *Ode: Intimations of Immortality from Recollections of Childhood*, a poem that idealizes the natural innocence and beauty of childhood

> was arguably as powerful an influence on nineteenth-century ideas of childhood as Freud has been on present day ones. The lines that we are born 'trailing clouds of glory' and that 'Heaven lies about us in our infancy' were repeatedly quoted, plagiarized and adapted by later writers.
>
> (ibid.: 27)

This outlook stood as a stark challenge to the reality of life for most children and the contradiction provided the basis for the campaigns to control and eventually end child labour, which ran through the nineteenth century. The various Factory Acts set limits to children's working hours and controlled the minimum age of work. The view began to take hold that even in the free-market laissez-faire atmosphere of Victorian politics it was possible to argue that the state should intervene to limit what businesses did in this area (Briggs 1999).

The state's sense of duty to children was paralleled by a growth of child-related philanthropy and charitable initiatives, many based on a sense of religious mission. Initiatives like Coram's foundling hospital grew and were joined by other institutions, such as Barnardo's in 1870 (Pugh 2007).

The idea underpinning the Romantic idea of childhood as a special phase of life was most obviously vindicated in the late nineteenth century by the development of compulsory state schooling. Gradually, the enforcement of compulsory attendance began to end the natural acceptance of the inevitability of children working. However, for a long time there remained a reluctance to accept the superior authority of the 'school board' or the truancy officer where children, especially older girls, were 'needed at home' (Hendrick 1997). As Heywood argues, 'The virtual elimination of the full-time employment of children in the developed economies of the West was a protracted process' (2001: 27).

By the beginning of the twentieth century there had emerged a clear idea of child-centredness in discussions about the family. Although the lives of most children were still dominated by poverty, ignorance and illness, a particular idea of the link between family relationships and the development of happy and healthy children had begun to take root, paving the way for the twentieth century, described by many commentators as 'the century of the child'.

The twentieth century: century of the child?

It is impossible to understand the changes in the view of children which developed in the twentieth century, without taking into account the growth of deliberate limitation of family size (Banks 1968). The spread of family limitation from the Victorian middle class to the rest of the population was a gradual process, which extended throughout the period up to the 1970s. What it led to was the decline in the average number of children per family from five or six in the 1870s to below two in the 1970s. This also needs to be considered in the light of the dramatic decline in infant mortality. Without accepting the view that high infant mortality inevitably correlates with parental indifference or lack of affection, it is clear that the decline in average family size had an influence on the extent to which time, effort and attention were devoted to individual children. One or two children are easier to focus on and idealize than eight or nine.

Schooling also creates a period of ambiguous status for children. The period of compulsory schooling, gradually extended throughout the twentieth century, is a time when children are not physically dependent on adults, yet they are not adults themselves. From nursery school to their late teens, children occupy a kind of limbo status with confused signals about rights and responsibilities offered at every turn. What is implicit in the provision of schooling, school health services, school dinners and so on, is the fact that this is a time when they are in need of protection, nurturing and guidance. Further, it is clear in the twentieth century that the welfare of children is not just a family responsibility. Children are seen as increasingly the responsibility of the state, which intervenes in their education, their health, their diet and their upbringing in ways designed to improve the national well-being by developing its future citizens. As Cunningham argues, one of the effects of two world wars in the UK was to produce '... a welfare state in which children were of central concern. Rarely has there been such a close identification between childhood and the destiny of the nation' (2006: 178).

A further development in the twentieth century is the idea of the child and their development as a proper subject for scientific study. The growth of psychology as a discipline is closely tied to the role it played in the increased surveillance and control of childhood, from IQ testing to identifying the origins of delinquency. As the century went on parents were bombarded with advice, often contradictory, on the appropriate ways to look after children. From Truby-King's regimented view of the importance of timing and routine, to the more relaxed perspectives of Benjamin Spock, there was a general view that the care and nurturing of children was a skilled task and not one which came naturally to parents through instinct (Hardyment 2007).

Childhood: what is it?

In this sense, however valid the criticisms levelled at Ariès and his colleagues may be, it does make sense to see our current notion of childhood as a modern invention. Primarily because of the spread of the middle-class ideology of the child-centred family, the development of compulsory universal schooling and the preoccupation of policy makers and welfare institutions with the interests of the child, there has come into being in the late twentieth century in the affluent West a different idea of childhood. This is a new and separate conception of childhood, which would have made little sense to our ancestors.

Student reflection

Does the suggestion that the concept of childhood as we know it did not exist before the seventeenth century necessarily imply that parents in bygone times did not love or care for their children?

This is not to say, of course, that children are not still abused, exploited and brutalized in the affluent West as well as elsewhere. Millions of children still live in poverty in the heart of affluent Europe and America. For much of the developing world the realities of child labour, high infant mortality, brutalization and enforced conscription of child soldiers, abandonment and exploitation remain facts of everyday life and make a mockery of earnest manifestos like the UN Declaration on the Rights of the Child (UN 1989). Similarly, the growing sense of children's rights has highlighted areas like sexual and physical abuse, which cast doubt on the idealistic image of a nurturing family. However, these failures and abuses are seen as contradicting the central value systems of the societies where they happen. Groups like UNICEF, the Child Poverty Action Group or Save the Children can appeal to the public's sense of what childhood *ought to be* like when they try to combat these problems. In this sense our idea of what it is to be a child is a social construct of modernity and one that affects all who are involved with children.

Key points

- Traditional approaches to history have largely neglected children.
- According to Ariès (1960) the concept childhood came into existence from the seventeenth century, driven mainly by the advance of universal schooling.
- Many social historians, including Ariès, follow the *sentiments* approach which states that from the seventeenth century there was a change in feelings and emotions towards children, from neutrality to high valuation.
- The work of Ariès and his followers has been criticized by others due to its theoretical and generalized nature and its use of evidence such as paintings and religious sermons, rather than the real experience of people as recorded in diaries and autobiographies.
- A dichotomy developed between the seventeenth-century Puritan and the nineteenth-century Romantic view of the child as innately sinful or innately pure, respectively.
- Nineteenth-century industrialization resulted in both the exploitation of child labour and the growing sense of duty to protect children coming from governments and philanthropic charities and individuals.
- The Romantic view of childhood took hold and, with the gradual development of compulsory state education, paved the way for the twentieth-century view of the child and the child-centred family.

- Today childhood is perceived not just as the responsibility of the family, but also of society and the state and is associated with the future prosperity of the nation. In other words, it is indeed a social construct of modernity.

Recommended reading

Ariès, P. (1960) *Centuries of Childhood*, Harmondsworth: Penguin Books.
Cunningham, H. (2006) *The Invention of Childhood*, London: BBC.
Orme, N. (2001) *Medieval Children*, New Haven: Yale University Press.
Rousseau, J.-J. (1911) [1762] *Emile*, London: Dent. Available online at: http://projects.ilt.columbia.edu/pedagogies/Rousseau/

References

Anderson, M. (1995) *Approaches to the History of the Western Family 1500–1914*, Cambridge: Cambridge University Press.
Ariès, P. (1960) *Centuries of Childhood*, Harmondsworth: Penguin Books.
Banks, J. A. (1968) *Prosperity and Parenthood*, London: Routledge and Kegan Paul.
Briggs, A. (1999) *England in the Age of Improvement*, London: Folio.
Cox, R. (1996) *Shaping Childhood: Themes of Uncertainty in the History of Adult–Child Relationships*, London: Routledge.
Cunningham, H. (2006) *The Invention of Childhood*, London: BBC.
De Mause, L. (ed.) (1995) *The History of Childhood*, New York: Aronson.
Dickens, C. (1971) [1837] *Oliver Twist*, Harmondsworth: Penguin Books.
Evans, R. J. (1997) *In Defence of History*, Granta: London.
Hardyment, C. (2007) *Dream Babies: Child Care from Locke to Spock*, London: Frances Lincoln.
Hendrick, H. (1994) *Child Welfare: England 1872–1989*, London: Longman.
—— (1997) *Children, Childhood and English Society, 1880–1990*, Cambridge: Cambridge University Press.
Heywood, C. (2001) *A History of Childhood*, Cambridge: Polity.
Kingsley, C. (1984) [1863] *The Water Babies*, Harmondsworth: Penguin Books.
McClure, R. K. (1981) *Coram's Children: The London Foundling Hospital in the Eighteenth Century*, London: Routledge.
Orme, N. (2001) *Medieval Children*, New Haven: Yale University Press.
Ozment, S. (1983) *When Fathers Ruled: Family Life in Reformation Europe*, Cambridge, MA: Harvard University Press.
Pollock, L. H. (1983) *Forgotten Children: Parent–Child Relations from 1500 to 1900*, Cambridge: Cambridge University Press.
Porter, R. (1990) *England in the Eighteenth Century*, London: Folio.
Pugh, G. (2007) *London's Forgotten Children: Thomas Coram and the Foundling Hospital*, Stroud: Tempus.
Rousseau, J.-J. (1979) [1762] *Emile*. Translated by Allan Bloom. New York: Basic Books.
Rowbotham, S. (1977) *Hidden from History: 300 Years of Women's Oppression and the Fight Against It*, 3rd edn, London: Pluto Classic.
Schama, S. (1987) *The Embarrassment of Riches: An Interpretation of Dutch Culture in the Golden Age*, London: Fontana.
Shahar, S. (1992) *Childhood in the Middle Ages*, London: Routledge.
Shorter, E. (1976) *The Making of the Modem Family*, London: Fontana.
Stone, L. (1977) *The Family, Sex and Marriage in England 1500–1800*, London: Weidenfeld.
Thompson, E. P. (1963) *The Making of The English Working Class*, London: Gollancz.
United Nations (UN) (1989) *Convention on the Rights of the Child*, New York: UN.

1.2 Construction of childhood
The building blocks

Shirley J. Pressler

Introduction

What do we mean by childhood? In a close examination of the history of Western childhood, Cunningham (1995) reveals that contemporary (Western) childhood has been viewed to be distinct from adulthood since the eighteenth century. However, Cunningham also states that this distinction has been bordering on change since the latter half of the twentieth century. Therefore, conceptualizations of Western childhood may be said to be in a state of tension, or to be undergoing transition. In this respect, Cunningham (1995) still provides a very useful framework for a discussion of our contemporary constructions of childhood:

> The peculiarity of the late twentieth century, and the root cause of much present confusion and angst about childhood, is that a public discourse which argues that children are persons with rights to a degree of autonomy is at odds with the remnants of the romantic view that the right of the child is to be a child. The implication of the first is a fusing of the worlds of adult and child, and the second the maintenance of separation.
>
> (ibid.: 190)

The Western construction of childhood presented here as being quite separate, or distant, from adulthood still remains, with perhaps some dissolution in sight. In terms of what is responsible for this separateness Cunningham makes reference to a Romantic view, in which he is alluding to the belief in childhood innocence. The public discourse he refers to is the relatively new children's rights discourse, which incorporates rights of provision, protection and participation (Alderson 2005; Burr 2004; Burr and Montgomery 2003; James and Prout 1997). Cunningham also makes reference to 'autonomy' as well as 'angst' and 'confusion', which implies an uneasy and complex construction of childhood. This complexity necessitates some exploration of childhood beyond Western constructions (Owusu-Bempah and Howitt 2000) and some thinking around the maintenance of *containment* (Jenks 2005), *inequity* (Burman 2008) and the associated notion of *toxicity* (Palmer 2006).

Containment here refers to the function of control and regulation imposed on children and young people, especially within education. *Inequity* really highlights the function of certain disadvantages, for example, social class and gender. *Toxicity* largely relates to the function, or by-products, of culturally driven mass-scale consumerism. The integration of extensions beyond Western constructions and these functions advocates some focus on, and revision of, childhood.

Within this chapter we will consider how images or concepts of childhood are constructed. We will firstly explore the adult–child distinction, or construction, from an experiential perspective. This will emphasize two things: first, the importance of socio-historical and socio-cultural contexts and second, the importance of the process of self-reflection. The first has a direct relationship with traditional and more contemporary constructions of childhood, while the latter has a direct relationship with pertinent issues raised by Owusu-Bempah and Howitt (2000), with special reference to how any of us construct childhood, essentially from a 'self'-restricting perspective. This is followed by an overview of prominent images and models of childhood, both the traditional ones commonly held responsible for the childhood–adulthood distinction, alongside the more contemporary ones related to the period of transition – hence incorporating the policy approach to childhood. Finally, a discussion of some of the consequences of traditional and contemporary constructions, as well as some more obscure constructions is undertaken.

The separate worlds of childhood and adulthood

A key question to consider when analysing childhood construction is: Where does adulthood start and where does childhood end?

Activity 1.2.1: The limits of childhood

The question above implies that the world of childhood is quite separate from that of adulthood.

- Take a few minutes to consider the key question above in relation to your own experience, jotting down any obvious points that spring to mind.

If you live in the UK you may have noted that this was marked by your 18th or 21st birthday, probably the former for younger people and the latter for people of more mature years. You may well have had fairly elaborate celebrations. You may have felt the pressure of a change in expectations from those around you, perhaps leading to much greater independence and responsibility, and a moving away from dependency and freedom from responsibility. Some of these pressures may have been permissions of law, for example, the responsibility to vote in general elections, or to take your driving test. However, in some parts of the world this transition, although similarly marked by rituals, appears quite different, and is often accompanied by an expectation of interdependence rather than independence (Penn 2005). Interestingly, Nelson Mandela recalls the time he experienced the marker of circumcision in his life, establishing his recognized change from child to adult, as is normal practice for the Xhosa tribe in South Africa where he grew up. His reflections usefully illustrate the culturally driven change from childhood to adulthood. While recounting the end of the period of seclusion he actively participated in with his peers, accommodated by the burial and burning of symbolic parts of his childhood, he writes:

> ... a lost and delightful world, the world of my childhood, the world of sweet and irresponsible days at Qunu and Mqhekezweni. Now I was a man, and I would never again play *thinti*, or steal maize, or drink milk from a cow's udder. I was already in

mourning for my own youth. Looking back, I know that I was not a man that day and would not truly become one for many years.

(Mandela 1995: 36)

We must consider whether this distinction between childhood and adulthood is a natural state of affairs or whether the distinction is a fabrication of the world we live in. The illustrations above do appear to confirm that the distinction is a fabrication, but that we may fall foul of accepting this distinction as natural, especially where we largely associate it with age. Although Mandela records that this transition happened when he was 16 years old, the testing yet meaningful ritual associated with symbolic artefacts was conducted over a period of time, and it was this, rather than age per se, that was deemed necessary in order for him to fully participate in society as a man. Where markers are associated with specific ages they are often decided on an arbitrary basis. In other words, we could decide any age in reality, which is perhaps why you can illogically marry with parental consent at 16 years of age, but only vote in a general election when you have reached 18 years of age in the UK. In the case of voting, here it is important to stress that this means that a person is actually disallowed from voting until they are 18 years of age. It is worth considering at this stage that one consequence of this involves exclusion from participating in this particular, seemingly democratic, process prior to age 18 simply on the basis of age in years, reflecting a lack of status rather than anything to do with ability, or competence (see James 1999; James and Prout 1997). The status of children and young people in relation to permissions of responsibility raises questions due to the trade-off between participatory rights and the protectionist rights associated with the Romantic notion of innocence. The importance of exclusion, from participation and democracy, which actually exemplify a separate world approach, may underlie much of the 'angst' and 'confusion' referred to by Cunningham (1995), but in essence denies the young person's participatory rights.

Overall, this separate child–adult world appears in part to arise from ideas about childhood, or certain discourses of childhood, evidenced in underlying images and models associated with them. While these appear to originate in philosophical considerations of personhood, or childhood, they are evident in historical accounts of childhood (Cunningham 1995) and can be seen in paintings and poetry (Montgomery 2003), children's literature, television advertisements, films and other media (Wyze 2004); charity advertising photographs (Burman 2008; Kehily and Montgomery 2003; Roche 2004) and family albums (Trafi 2008); advice leaflets (Burman 1994; 2008); as well as in academic writing more generally.

Images and models of childhood

An image or a model is not a simply a picture. An image is a repeated general representation from a sequence of pictures across various forms of media and across extended periods of history. When considering images and models used to construct perceptions of childhood, Holland (2004: 3–4) refers to resonant images. She describes a resonant image as a key public image reflected repeatedly through different pictures, creating a typology and meaning in the collective public consciousness. She goes on to state that resonant images are dependent on socio-cultural and historical factors, so changes in images can reveal changes in social thinking and vice versa. Activity 1.2.2 below asks you to consider a photograph in order to arrive at one of the traditional resonant images of childhood.

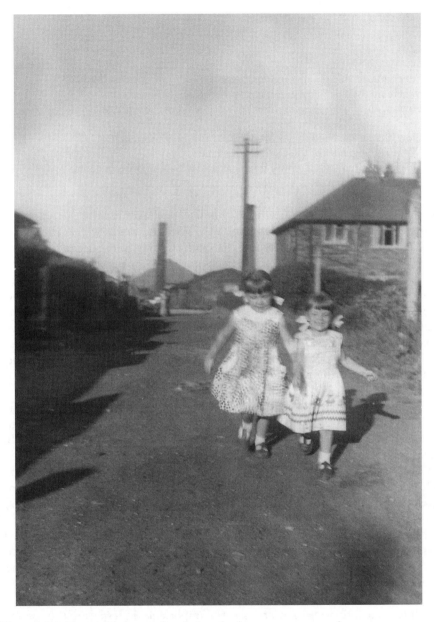

Figure 1.2.1 Two children running down a backstreet on a sunny day.

Activity 1.2.2: Reading photographs

Study the photograph above (Figure 1.2.1) for a few minutes, then answer the following questions.

- When might this photograph have been taken?
- Where might this photograph have been taken?
- How wealthy were these children, or what kind of class do these children come from (working, middle or privileged)?
- How old are the children and why might this be important?
- What is the gender of the children depicted?
- Do the children look happy and look as if they have relative freedom?

Let us consider our possible response to the picture above. Firstly, this photograph is obviously quite dated. We can tell this from the surroundings as well as the clothes that the children are wearing. We can assume that both children were born in the mid-1950s. Secondly, the photograph was clearly taken somewhere in the industrialized Western world; there are noticeable clues in the photograph. You may have guessed that it was taken in the UK, in the North West. Thirdly, these children do not look particularly privileged, nor do they look absolutely poor. They do not appear particularly middle-class, certainly not by their surroundings. If you guessed working-class then you were correct. However, they do look healthy, are well groomed, clean and appear well looked after. This contrasts with some images of working-class children who are commonly shown in relation to poverty during this particular era, for example, those depicted by Dudgeon and Cox (2001).

The children seem to have been about three and four years of age at the time the photograph was taken and both are girls. We can make all types of assumptions regarding the implications that their gender may have had for them, particularly during this era, or at and from this point in history.

The photograph can be said to position these particular children in a particular socio-historical and cultural context. Bearing socio-historical cultural contexts in mind is extremely important because it aids our understanding of diverse childhoods; both within as well as between cultures. We can guess that both children attended school from around 5 years of age. However, if the photograph had been taken at a date prior to the universal schooling of children in the UK (1872 according to Penn 2005), we would not necessarily make the same assumption. Regardless of date we might not make the same assumption elsewhere in the world.

While all these answers might give us some indication of the kind of lives these particular children led, they also concern issues of importance in respect of the construction of resonant images childhood. This is where the last question in Activity 1.2.1 becomes particularly important as it alludes to a particular construction, or image, of childhood.

Childhood as a time of innocence

The children in the photograph appear to be happy, are skipping along and thus appear relatively carefree. This interpretation is aided by the fact that the children appear to be surrounded by sunshine in the photograph. This particular image of childhood has special significance in the Western world, since it involves an image of childhood as a time of innocence, one stemming from the Romantic notion of childhood as portrayed by Rousseau in *Emile*, first published in 1762 (translated 1979). The resonant image is of an idyllic childhood, one of freedom and exploration, a time to be happy and carefree, without responsibilities. The child is conceptualized as inherently or naturally good and ideally free from adult oppression, especially in an educational setting (Montgomery 2003). (For an interesting discussion about the 'public' and 'private' aspects of such photographs see Trafi 2008.) It is argued that in some cultures the belief in childhood innocence is partly responsible for the separation of childhood from adulthood, particularly in relation to status, and hence treatment, of children in contemporary society (James 1999; Jenks 2005).

Exploring constructions of childhood: discourses, images and models

There are generally considered to be three models or resonant images of childhood – the angelic, the demonic and the small person model. These images are aligned with three sets of discourse, or areas of language use in relation to children, which in fact construct the images – the Romantic, the Puritan and the Rights-based discourses (Alderson 2005).

Rousseau's Romantic view of the child, or Romantic discourse, where the child is constructed as innocent, is aligned with the idea that children naturally develop, in accordance with the theoretical perspective of Piaget (Piaget and Inhelder 1969) as well as with *child-centred* approaches in practice (Burman 2008). The theory is held responsible for constructing childhood as a time of neediness, thus requiring protection. Woodhead (2003: 120), labelling this as a 'developmentalism' discourse, asserts that this view constructs the child as not yet an adult and in the process of becoming a person in her/his own right.

In contrast, Hobbes's Puritan view, or Puritan discourse, where the child is constructed to be wicked or evil, is generally aligned with the need for shaping and regulation. In a sense, the child is also constructed through this image as being incomplete or 'unwhole'. According to Jenks (2005), childhood associated with the Puritan discourse has escalated since the murder of a young child by two other children as a result of the two children digressing from the construction of childhood associated with the Romantic discourse. This is expanded upon below.

Montgomery (2003) discusses research in which parents were interviewed about their own, as well as their children's, childhood:

> While examining daily patterns of child rearing, she [Ribbens] asked parents how they conceptualized their children. … However, the constructions of children as angelic, corrupt, devilish or innocent have a history in Western thought, and their influence can still be seen today. It is interesting to discover whether these philosophical discourses that Ribbens mentions – children as small people – will become more important in parents' lives.
>
> (ibid.: 67)

In contrast to the Romantic and the Puritan discourses, Montgomery notes that, while parental constructions were implicit rather than explicit, the research found that parents did not 'talk about children as incomplete beings becoming adults'. Moreover, while the parents varied in their constructions of childhood, as associated with either innocence, wickedness or children being (small) people, the research suggested that indeed these images do to some extent align with the Romantic, Puritan and Rights-based discourses and they do not assume a needs-driven or half-people (Alderson 2005) approach.

Problematized and negative constructions of childhood

The belief in inherent wickedness is one in keeping with the Puritan discourse of childhood. Proponents of this view hold a construction of childhood as uncivilized, one exemplified in Golding's (1954) book *Lord of the Flies* where, left to their own devices, a group of boys resort to savagery.

Both the Puritan discourse and the 'tabula rasa' discourse, with an inherent 'blank slate' construction of the child, position childhood as 'a time of becoming'. This results in parents and educators being held responsible for controlling innate savagery and producing rational civilized beings (Montgomery 2003).

The Bulger case

In 1993, the killing of two-year-old James Bulger in Liverpool in the UK by two ten-year-old boys enhanced the Puritan image of the child as innately evil and incited the public to call for the reinstatement of the death penalty: 'As the boys were taken to court a mob gathered outside the courtroom screaming for them to be given the death penalty' (Kehily 2004: 16).

Jenks (2005) considers that the Bulger case was pivotal to contemporary images of childhood. He suggests that children who do not conform to the resonant Romantic notion of innocence held by adults, and deviate from this image, as did the two ten year olds in the Bulger case, are held to be wicked. Both boys in this case were tried as adults at an age when in many countries they would not have been held legally accountable, and both received sentences which excluded them from society for a long period of time.

In a similar case in Norway, the child killers, deemed not to be legally accountable for their action, were reintegrated into society, and were accompanied by psychologists for some time. The mother of the young girl who was murdered in Norway expressed a view that differed quite sharply from that of the screaming mob in the UK. She appeared to rationalize that the children did not fully understand the consequences of their actions, even if they did have some realization about what they did and she accepted their reintegration into society (Montgomery 2003).

The treatment of childhood: justice versus welfare

The difference in treatment of the child killers in the two cases mentioned above appears to reflect the *justice* versus *welfare* models of the treatment of children raised by Asquith, as discussed by Stainton Rogers (2003). The justice and welfare models respectively align with the Puritan and the Romantic discourses. It is interesting to note that a justice orientation is one ascribed to by a masculine stance and the care orientation, implicit in the welfare model, is one ascribed to by a feminine stance in Gilligan's (1982) critique of the order of Kohlberg's levels of moral reasoning (Kohlberg 1980). Thus the justice orientation may be more aligned with the patriarchal structure of society, while the care orientation more with feminist concerns.

Arguably, the justice orientation has greater alliance with objectivism and distant ways of relating, those favoured by scientific regulation and control, and an individualistic stance. This worldview is in keeping with valuing and fostering competitiveness, and consequently, inequity. On the other hand, the care orientation has arguably greater alliance with subjectivism and essentially merged ways of relating, those favoured by social constructionist visions of acceptance of diversity, deregulation and a collectivist stance. This is a worldview in keeping with valuing and fostering co-operation, and consequently, equity. These contrasting worldviews are related to the differing goals of development evident in individualistic and collectivist societies (Burman 1999; Penn 2005), those associated with fostering an independent versus an interdependent sense of self (Alderson 2005; Owusu-Bempah and Howitt 2000).

The discussion above would suggest that the treatment of children in the UK is aligned with a justice orientated, masculine worldview based on competition and harbouring and propagating inequality, and that this worldview is shaped frequently by Puritan discourses about childhood.

On 3 October 2008 the BBC News showed images of hooded youths wandering around in a group seemingly misbehaving. At the same time it was announced that the prevalence of such images and the negativity associated with them were condemned by the UN in a report released on the same day (UN, 2008). The report highlights the over-prevalence of such negative images and accords this with the inappropriate negative treatment of young people in the UK. It emphasizes that such images along with the high prevalence of locking up young people, at a greater rate than any other in Europe, and the prevalence of poverty, along with the use of Anti-Social Behaviour Orders (ASBOs) and mosquito devices, breach the human rights of children and young people. The news item featured a youth, who had been incarcerated for burglary and misdemeanours, being interviewed. When asked about incarceration, he stated that being locked up was of no benefit and in his view did nothing to help or change behaviour. He added that, as in his case, there were reasons why people did unacceptable things and that these reasons needed to be listened to. In his view it was the latter that was more beneficial to helping and changing behaviour. This young man appeared polite, articulate, reasonable and highly rational.

This case study reflects concerns raised by academic writers in relevant contemporary literature already referred to. It emphasizes the need to listen to young people, especially when they appear to transgress, and especially when considering the reasons for apparent transgressions. The transgressions noted in the UK may well be the product of, or duplication of, the world that young people experience. This is supported by research that takes a non-objectification stance (Grieg and Taylor 1999), one which ascribes to the notion of children being social actors in their own rights (Kehily and Swann 2003; Woodhead 2004). This approach alerts us to the duplication of hierarchical power struggles in relation to adult–child relationships as well as to gender relationships. Moreover, this research focuses on 'voicing' the experiences of young people within families, schools and the community in contemporary society (Cullingford 2007).

Traditional developmental psychology: toxicity, containment and inequality

Previous reports have declared that youth in the UK are both the unhappiest and the worst behaved in Europe. Lifestyle and the pace of life contribute to a construction of childhood culminating in a form Palmer (2006) terms 'toxicity'. Jenks (2005) uses the term 'containment' to refer to the treatment of children, especially within education, and partly attributes this to the pivotal Bulger case and pace of life. Burman (2008) uses a construction of 'inequity' when describing the treatment of children, especially in relation to gender and class.

It could be suggested that these negative facets of the treatment of children and the constructions of childhood within our contemporary society – toxicity, containment and inequality – are in part attributable to traditional developmental psychology and to the prevalence of both the Romantic and the Puritan discourses of childhood.

Both Jenks (2005) and Burman (2008) subscribe to the view that traditional developmental psychology contributes much to these unhappy positions by way of constructing the child as in a process of becoming. Thus children are generally perceived of as immature, and seen as following a natural development aligned with a Romantic discourse – unless there is some deviation from the expected Romantic trajectory, in which case they are constructed through a Puritan discourse. These inherent features of Piagetian theory have an aim, or end point, of a civilized rational being.

Stainton Rogers (2004) also appears to subscribe to the condemnation of developmental psychology. In respect of the needs discourse, she lays responsibility at the feet of outdated policy as well as developmental psychology, but does not reflect on the latter as outdated. Penn (2005) makes a valuable point about the use of outdated developmental psychology, one which has some overlap with Woodhead's varied views of developmental psychology, as expressed by Woodhead (1997; 2004) (see above).

In defence of Piagetian developmental psychology, it could be suggested that many childhood textbooks simply align Piaget's theories with developmental psychology and age-stage related development and through (mis)application of the theory position the child as passive. Piaget's theory actually constructs the child as active and as such might be usefully aligned with matters pertaining to participatory rights.

Well-being, the quality of life discourse and future projections

Some deliberation needs to be undertaken with the aim of moving towards a more positive construction of childhood, one which is more constructive and enabling than the negative and destructive construction discussed.

In order to do so we may need to look to lifespan approaches and contemporary developmental psychology. The remit of contemporary developmental psychology advocates participation, competencies, positive aspects of digression, multidirectional change across the lifespan and socio-historical and cultural contexts, including 'synchronicity' from a nested systems approach (see Figure 1.2.2). Sugarman (2001) considers treatment approaches and Mufti (2006) considers approaches in education that have implications for psychological well-being. Each implies a move towards the 'fusion' referred to by Cunningham (1995) by way of merged perspective taking, similar to those currently acknowledged in children's literature (Hunt 2004; Kehily 2004) and with relevance in respect of arguments offered by Owusu-Bempah and Howitt (2000). Such considerations are especially important during an era of the introduction of academies and the consideration of extending the age of compulsory education.

But childhood prolonged cannot remain a fairyland. It becomes a hell.
— Louise Bogan (1897–1970)

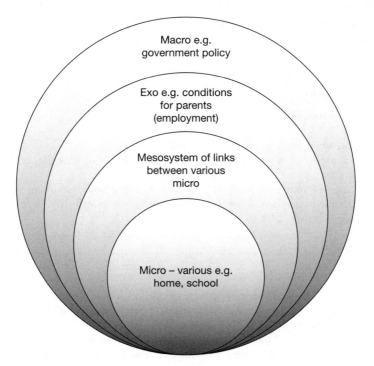

Figure 1.2.2 Nested systems approach representing the Ecological Model (adapted from Smith *et al.* 2003).

Activity 1.2.3: Media representations

Select a variety of articles about children and young people, preferably from different sources, such as a newspaper, a parenting magazine and a magazine for young people.
   Read through the articles several times, reviewing and analysing them as you do so. Consider how the children and young people are constructed.

- Are they positioned as a threat, compliant, needy or socially active in their own right? Can you see implicit evidence for the Puritan, 'tabula rasa', Romantic or Rights-based discourses?
- What, if any, treatment approaches are implied in the articles? Are these 'justice' or 'welfare' oriented?

Discuss your analysis with a friend, partner, colleague or fellow student.

Conclusion

Future conceptualizations of childhood need to move away from traditional developmental psychology and both the Romantic and Puritan discourses. We must focus on the inclusion and participatory aspects of life and, most importantly, we must seek to construct images of childhood that constitute children as people, not as becoming people, through a Rights-based discourse. Debates considering the quality of life discourse need to move towards appreciating research that informs a more positive construction of childhood, including that informed by the reality of the lived experiences voiced by children themselves, as well as the reality constructed by their parents.

Student reflection

Consider your own childhood:

- When and where were you born and raised?
- What was expected of you at different age-related stages of your life, or due to your gender?
- What image of your childhood do you hold? Is this a nostalgic image containing a view of a time of freedom to roam and freedom from responsibility?
- What role did adults play in your life?

Key points

- Contemporary Western societies perceive of childhood as separate from adulthood and construct childhood as a period of becoming (a person or an adult). This view is not shared by all cultures.
- Resonant images of childhood in contemporary Western societies have been constructed from sets of pictures and images across different media and across time, and are dependent on socio-cultural, historical and political factors.
- There are three generalized models or images of childhood in Western societies – angelic, demonic and small person – and these are aligned respectively to three discourse sets – the Romantic, the Puritan and the Rights-based.
- The James Bulger case in the UK in 1993 added to the demonic image of childhood espoused by the Puritan discourse.
- The treatment of the child killers in this case suggests that in the UK the treatment of children is frequently aligned to a justice orientated, competitive, masculine worldview based on Puritan discourse which propagates inequality.
- In a sense, both the Romantic and Puritan discourses construct childhood as a process of becoming (people or adults) in line with traditional developmental psychology.
- Both discourses, therefore, in line with traditional developmental psychology, construct negative images of children based on concepts of dependency, moral immaturity and need for containment and protection from toxicity, both societal and self-induced.
- For this reason many would advocate a contemporary developmental psychology approach to childhood which focuses on listening to and including children's voices and perceiving children as participants in society as people, not as becoming people.

Recommended reading

Kirby, P. and Woodhead, M. (2003) Children's participation in society, in H. Montgomery, R. Burr and M. Woodhead (eds) *Changing Childhoods: Local and Global*, Chichester: John Wiley/OU.

Newman, M. (2006) When evidence is not enough: freedom to choose versus prescribed choice: the case of Summerhill School, in D. Kassem, E. Mufti and J. Robinson (eds) *Education Studies: Issues and Critical Perspectives*, Maidenhead: McGraw-Hill/OUP.

Sanders, B. (2004) Childhood in different cultures, Chapter 5 in T. Maynard and N. Thomas (eds) *An Introduction to Early Childhood Studies*, London: Sage.

References

Alderson, P. (2005) Children's rights: a new approach to studying childhood, in H. Penn, *Understanding Early Childhood: Issues and Controversies*, Maidenhead: McGraw-Hill/OUP.

BBC News (2008) Children's rights 'ignored'. Available online at: http://news.bbc.co.uk/go/em/fr/-/1/hi/uk/7652098.stm (accessed 5 October 2008).

—— Children's rights 'not being met'. Available online at: http://news.bbc.co.uk/go/em/fr/-/1/hi/uk/7651184.stm (accessed 5 October 2008).

Burman, E. (1994) *Deconstructing Developmental Psychology*, London: Routledge.

—— (1999) Morality and the goals of development, in M. Woodhead, D. Faulkner and K. Littleton (eds), *Making Sense of Social Development*, London: Routledge.

—— (2008) *Deconstructing Developmental Psychology*, 2nd edn, London: Routledge.

Burr, R. (2004) Children's rights: international policy and lived practice, in M. J. Kehily (ed.) *An Introduction to Childhood Studies*, Berkshire: McGraw-Hill.

Burr, R. and Montgomery, H. (2003) Children and rights, in M. Woodhead and H. Montgomery (eds) *Understanding Childhood: An Interdisciplinary Approach*, Chichester: John Wiley/OU.

Cullingford, C. (2007) *Childhood – The Inside Story: Hearing Children's Voices*, Newcastle: Cambridge.

Cunningham, H. (1995) *Children and Childhood in Western Society since 1500*, London: Longman.

Dudgeon, P. and Cox, J. (2001) *Josephine Cox Child of the North: Memories of a Northern Childhood*, London: Hodder Headline.

Gilligan, C. (1982) *In a Different Voice: Psychological Theory and Women's Development*, Cambridge, MA: Harvard University Press.

Golding, W. (1962) [1954] *Lord of the Flies*, London: Faber.

Greig, A. and Taylor, J. (1999) *Doing Research with Children*, London: Sage.

Holland, P. (2004) *Picturing Childhood: The Myth of the Child in Popular Imagery*. London: I. B. Tauris.

Hunt, P. (2004) Children's literature and childhood, in M. J. Kehily (ed.) *An Introduction to Childhood Studies*, Berkshire: McGraw-Hill.

James, A. (1999) Researching children's social competence: methods and models, in M. Woodhead, D. Faulkner and K. Littleton (eds) *Making Sense of Social Development*, London: Routledge/OU.

James, A. and Prout, A. (eds) (1997) *Constructing and Reconstructing Childhood: Contemporary Issues in the Sociological Study of Childhood*, 2nd edn, London: Falmer Press.

Jenks, C. (2005) *Childhood*, 2nd edn, Abingdon: Routledge.

Kehily, M. J. (2004) Understanding childhood: an introduction to some key themes and issues, in M. J. Kehily (ed.) *An Introduction to Childhood Studies*, Berkshire: McGraw-Hill.

Kehily, M. J. and Montgomery, H. (2003) Innocence and experience, in M. Woodhead and H. Montgomery (eds) *Understanding Childhood: An Interdisciplinary Approach*, Chichester: John Wiley/OU.

Kehily, M. J. and Swann, J. (2003) *Children's Cultural Worlds*, Chichester: John Wiley/OU.

Kohlberg, L. (1980) *The Meaning and Measurement of Moral Development*, Worcester, MA: Clark University Press.

Mandela, N. (1995) *Long Walk to Freedom*, London: Abacus.

Montgomery, H. (2003) Childhood in time and place, in M. Woodhead and H. Montgomery (eds) *Understanding Childhood: An Interdisciplinary Approach*, Chichester: John Wiley/OU.

Mufti, E. (2006) New students: same old structures, in D. Kassem, E. Mufti and J. Robinson (eds) *Education Studies: Issues and Critical Perspectives*, Maidenhead: McGraw-Hill/OUP.

Nsamenang, A. B. and Lamb, M. E. (1998) Socialization of Nso children in the Bamenda grassfields of Northwest Cameroon, in M. Woodhead, D. Faulkner and K. Littleton (eds) *Cultural Worlds of Early Childhood*, London: Routledge/OU.

Owusu-Bempah, K. and Howitt, D. (2000) *Psychology Beyond Western Perspectives*, Leicester: BPS Books.

Palmer, S. (2006) *Toxic Childhood: How the Modern World is Damaging Our Children and What We Can Do about It*, London: Orion.

Penn, H. (2005) *Understanding Early Childhood: Issues and Controversies*, Maidenhead: McGraw-Hill/OUP.

Piaget, J. and Inhelder, B. (1969) *The Psychology of the Child*, New York: Basic Books.

Roche, P. (2004) *Unloved: The True Story of a Stolen Childhood*, London: Penguin.

Rousseau, J.-J. (1979) [1762] *Emile, or On Education*, translated by Alan Bloom, New York: Basic Books.

Smith, P. K., Cowie, H. and Blades, M. (2003) *Understanding Children's Development*, 4th edn, Oxford: Blackwell.

Stainton Rogers, W. (2003) What is a child? in M. Woodhead and H. Montgomery (eds) *Understanding Childhood: An Interdisciplinary Approach*, Chichester: John Wiley/OU.

—— (2004) Promoting better childhoods: constructions of child concern, in M. J. Kehily (ed.) *An Introduction to Childhood Studies*, Berkshire: McGraw-Hill.

Sugarman, L. (2001) *Lifespan Development: Frameworks, Accounts and Strategies*, 2nd edn, Hove: Psychology Press.

Trafi, L. (2008) A visual culture art education curriculum for early childhood teacher education: re-constructing the family album, *The International Journal of Art & Design Education*, 27 (1), 53–62.

UN (2008) Most recent concluding observations, United Kingdom of Great Britain and Northern Ireland and UN Treaty Bodies, Committee on the Rights of the Child. Available at http://www.ohchr.org/EN/Countries/ENACARegion/Pages/GBIndex.aspx

Woodhead, M. (1997) Psychology and the cultural construction of children's needs, in A. James and A. Prout (eds) *Constructing and Reconstructing Childhood: Contemporary Issues in the Sociological Study of Childhood*, 2nd edn, London: Falmer Press.

—— (2003) The child in development, in M. Woodhead and H. Montgomery (eds) *Understanding Childhood: An Interdisciplinary Approach*, Chichester: John Wiley/OU.

—— (2004) Foreword, in M. J. Kehily (ed.) *An Introduction to Childhood Studies*, Berkshire: McGraw-Hill.

Wyze, D. (ed.) (2004) *Childhood Studies: An Introduction*, Oxford: Blackwell.

1.3 Race, racism and mixed heritage

A mixed life

Derek Kassem

I love my mixed race baby – but why does she feel so alien?

— Lowri Turner (2007)

I consider you are not fit to bring up your daughter with your ideas of mating her to a Negro. I sincerely hope that God will cut short your life and that you will *die soon* so that dear little white girl may be saved from the hideous fate you plan for her. A black blubber-lipped Negro on top of her!

Interbreeding is evil and nobody could be proud of half-caste children. The idea of everyone being a wretched khaki colour with thick lips and flat noses in the future is abhorrent to all right-thinking Englishmen.

— Letters received by the Reverend Clifford Hill after a broadcast in 1961 during which he said that he would not object to his daughter marrying a black man quoted in Alibhai-Brown (2001: 1)

Introduction

Race and racism in Western society has been an ever-present force since the days of empire in which it was used to justify the dominance and subjugation of non-white peoples. As Ali (2002) points out, the great tragedies of history are often presented in a void. No explanation is offered and they are viewed as an inexplicable and incomprehensible act on the part of fanatical fundamentalists with no feelings. This representation of the events of 11 September 2001 in New York is also used to further justify the growth of racism and racist parties across Western Europe, along with the concomitant Islamophobia (Fekete 2009). That British society is racist is recognized both by the white indigenous community and the non-white communities that currently make up the multicultural society that is the UK. The Runnymede Trust (1992) found that 67 per cent of whites claimed that Britain was racist, and 79 per cent of blacks and 56 per cent of Asians agreed with the white population. The fact that the Runnymede survey of 1992 was some time ago and at that time there were no elected representatives of racist and fascist parties on local councils or other public bodies suggests that society and the body politic has travelled some distance in dealing with issues surrounding race, migration and specifically the

Islamic community. In many respects, the change has been fuelled by the events of 2001 and the subsequent tragedies that occurred in London and Madrid. As Fekete (2009) points out, current discourse from mainstream political parties forms a xeno-racism. What is meant by this term is the global nature of the driving forces of racism that are linked to the conflicts in Iraq and Afghanistan, along with issues of security, terrorism anti-migration and fortress Europe.

Just as it is not possible to understand an act of barbarity such as the events identified above, it is also not possible to understand the contradictions of the perceptions of race without examining the context in which they take place. The rise of hostility marked by the increased political prominence of racist parties and the frequent hostility of the mainstream parties' discourse aimed at, for instance, the Muslim community, has to be seen against the backdrop of increased interracial relationships between individuals (Asthana and Smith 2009).

Interracial relationships and the mixed-race individuals that they produce challenge many ideas about race and ethnicity that are held as common sense by many individuals. Their very existence challenges the idea of distinct races among the peoples of the world. Montagu (1997) in his book on the fallacy of race points out that:

> ... to make use of the scientifically established facts to show that the term race is a socially constructed artefact – that there is no such thing in reality as race, that the very word is racist; that the idea of race, implying the existence of significant biologically determined mental differences rendering some populations inferior to others, is wholly false; and that space between an idea and reality can be very great and misleading.
>
> (31)

That race is a social and cultural construct with no basis in biology is true, however, the emotions that race is capable of engendering are powerful and frequently destructive to society's well-being. This chapter is going to discuss the growth and development of the UK as an increasingly diverse society with specific reference to mixed-race individuals. Mixed-race individuals by their very nature come from a varied and diverse set of backgrounds but they do have something in common. They are a young group that are also one of the fastest-growing ethnic groups in the UK. Therefore, the issues that they face both as individuals and as a group, albeit a heterogeneous group, are the issues and problems that the UK will be facing in the future, for mixed-race children are a major part of the future of Britain.

Mixed-race populations

Britain is predominately mono-ethnic with a white British population that encompasses around 85 per cent of individuals belonging to this group (Platt 2009). The largest minority group within the UK is the Indian heritage community making up approximately 2 per cent of the population. The other main ethnic minority groups include: the Pakistani heritage community (1.6 per cent), Black Africans (1.2 per cent), Black Caribbeans (1 per cent), the Bangladeshi heritage commuinity (0.6 per cent) and the Chinese community (0.4 per cent) (ibid.). The mixed-race group, for the purpose of data collection, were defined in four different categories, which make up 1.1 per cent of the population combined (ibid.).

Activity 1.3.1: Ethnic minorities in the UK

Research the actual size of the ethnic minority population in the UK. Carry out a small survey asking people to estimate the size of the ethnic minority population.

- Do they over estimate, underestimate or give about the right answer?
- Can you explain some of the responses you received from your survey?

The size of the minority ethnic population in the UK is in fact quite small (see above) compared to the indigenous population. However, the demographic profile of the various minority groups is different from the majority population. The minority groups tend to be younger than the majority population (Owen 2001). One in five, or 20 per cent, of children under the age of 16 were from minority groups and 3 per cent of children under the age of 16 were identified as coming from a mixed-race background (Platt 2009). Furthermore, one in ten children in the UK now live in a mixed-race family (Asthana and Smith 2009). There is comparatively limited knowledge of the make-up of the mixed-race community as the identification and quantification of the nature and extent of mixed-race relationships were only officially recognized for the first time in the 2001 Census. The Census return identified approximately 674, 000 people as mixed-race. The demographers identified the mixed-race community as one of the fastest-growing of all ethnic groups within the UK. It should be pointed out that the mixed group only represent 1.3 per cent of the total population, however, this translates into just over 14 per cent of the ethnic minority population of the UK as a whole (Song 2007). It is estimated that by 2010 the numbers of mixed-race individuals will have increased by 40 per cent and by more than 80 per cent in the year 2020 (Song 2007).

Activity 1.3.2: Attitudes to mixed-race relationships

Carry out a small survey to find out individuals' attitudes to mixed-race relationships.

- Which relationships are acceptable, which are not?
- Can you explain the attitudes of the people you have surveyed?
- What do you think this tells you about community relationships in the UK?

The projected increase in the size of the mixed-race community needs to be taken with a great deal of caution, as there are problems of definition, which may underestimate the actual extent of the community in the first instance. The possible combinations identified as mixed-race in the Census, for instance, were comparatively narrow in scope. They were: 'White/Black Caribbean'; 'White/Black African'; 'White/Asian' and, a catch-all 'Any Other' mixed background. The problem with this categorization of 'mixedness' is that it does not allow for mixed-race individuals other than in terms of whiteness, a racist perspective in many ways. A Black Caribbean/Asian category, for example, was not provided except within the catch-all statement of 'Any Other'. Therefore, there is a lack of an accurate picture of the make-up of the mixed community. This lack of knowledge of the nature of mixed-race individuals also sets up challenges for the various ethnic minority communities and how they respond to the growth of interracial relationships.

It also needs to be recognized that the state is, in effect, defining the nature of 'mixed-race' through both the number of options and the form they take in major compulsory social surveys such as the Census (Aspinall 2003). The state-defined categories of acceptable combinations used to define mixed-race are then copied throughout government organizations and in the wider community – typically companies who want to be seen to be collecting data for equal opportunity purposes. The lack of official recognition can and does tend to lead to invisibility for a large number of mixed ethnic minority groups (Aspinall 2000). Consequently, the characteristics and the needs of the invisible are not supported through any government action or policy. This may have detrimental effects in areas such as education, health or any other relevant social need.

That mixed-race individuals are the product of interracial relationships is an obvious truism. The pattern of these relationships is of importance for the ethnic minority communities as much as the indigenous majority community. The extent of interracial relationships differs across different communities. For instance, ethnic minority men and women born in or mainly brought up in the UK are more likely to enter into an interracial relationship (Platt 2009), though men did tend to engage in higher levels of interracial relationships. Age is a key element in interracial relationships as the younger a person is the more likely they are to enter into interracial relationships and/or marriage (ibid.). The limitations of the development of interracial relationships are the relative size of the communities the individual lives in, and the established nature of, their community – that is the number of second and third generation individuals in the community.

Towards a definition of mixed-race

For many individuals the term 'mixed-race' is a very unsatisfactory term and is no more useful, or no less offensive, than the category of half-caste (Bellos 2007). The very notion of mixed-race has a limited applicability; it does not include, for example, a child of German/French parentage. This classification and other similar European combinations would not be defined as mixed-race. It is the inclusion of non-white that creates the idea of mixed-race. In fact, in common usage any combination of ethnic grouping that includes a black parent will result in a 'black' child (Gordon 2004). This suggests that the very idea of mixed-race is defined in terms of blackness with all the concomitant links to racism. The identity of the child is defined in terms of their relationship to colour, not in terms of any genuine notions of mixed heritage as culture is effectively ignored. In other words, ethnicity refers purely to the degree of blackness of the individual. This harks back to the old slave-owning societies, which defined levels of 'blackness' by the degree of 'blackness' back through generations.

For the individual concerned this view of mixed-race carries with it all the prejudices that black people meet plus the denial of their whole cultural and ethnic heritage. Individuals who are further removed from what might be termed black due to racial combinations including ethnic groups other than white, for example, Arab and Asian, are effectively ignored. Their existence is marginalized. Their identities and claims of cultural need are taken as irrelevant or just confused and mistaken by a white society which they are both a member of and not a member of simultaneously.

At the heart of the idea of mixed-race is racism that is imposed on individuals by white society, as Bellos (2007) states:

The need to describe oneself as mixed, or the desire of society to define us as such, is something which should be questioned. Let us not confuse the need to define our own identity with a rush to put us in a category which subtly but unmistakeably names us 'part black' as though it was a taint. If one parent or grandparent is African we are right to call ourselves African if we wish, but it should not be mandatory.

(27)

Activity 1.3.3: History of minority populations in the UK

Research the history of ethnic minority populations in the UK.

- When did the first Black and Asian people come to this country? It was not after the Second World War.
- What areas of the country did Black and Asian people first settle and why?
- Apart from Black and Asian communities, can you identify other ethnic minority groups that have settled in the UK and the reasons for their settlement?
- What does all the information you have researched tell you about the population of the UK?

The labelling of individuals in terms of their relationship to blackness denies the individual the right to their own identity as perceived by themselves as well as denying the mixed heritage of other individuals – the effective erasing of their individuality.

The experience of mixed race

The term 'mixed-race' is the most polite term used to describe an individual whose parents come from two different ethnic groups. The author, who is of mixed heritage (Egyptian/ Scottish), was once called 'nigger meat' by members of a neo-Nazi organization who parade as British nationalists. However, there are many other terms of abuse including half-caste, half-breed, wog, golly, jungle bunny etc. These insults come thick and fast in a racist society. These are terms of abuse that many children face on a daily basis in our school system, though surprisingly they occur more in primary schools than in secondary schools (Tizard and Phoenix 2002). Racist insults are aimed just as much at mixed-race pupils as at black or other ethnic minority pupils (ibid.). Racist name-calling is only part of the racist experience; racist stereotyping, differential treatment, straightforward discrimination and institutional racism all play their part in the mixed-race child's school days. These experiences have a direct impact on the levels of educational achievement by the different groups that make up the mixed-race community.

Tikly (2007) found that the attainment of White/Black Caribbean pupils is below average in primary and secondary schools. Of all the mixed groups, they underperformed to the greatest extent (Caballero, *et al.* 2007). White/African pupils, for instance, were near average as a group in terms of their levels of attainment at both primary and secondary levels. In the same study, a group identified as White/Asian were deemed to be performing academically above average. These findings clearly raise some important issues in terms of the academic performance of the groups but it also raises yet again the issue of definition. For example, what constitutes 'Asian'? There are many different ethnic and religious groups that come under the heading Asian. By drawing together such a diverse group and defining them in terms of their relationship to white, there is the real possibility that the data do not represent the true levels of achievement of significant groups of pupils. The same considerations also apply to White/African. It would be similar and just as nonsensical as using 'European' to describe 'white', as there are many different cultures in Europe. White always means the indigenous population: English, Scottish or Welsh. The Irish have been left out because there has been a history of discrimination against the Irish community within the UK.

All the issues that have been identified as applying to the black community within the education system, such as low teacher expectations, stereotyping, relatively high exclusion rates, apply to mixed-race pupils, especially those who are part Afro-Caribbean (Gillborn 2008). Tikly (2007) also points out that the pupil response is often to adopt a rebellious black identity with the appropriate behaviour patterns, thus he argues that this reinforces the teachers' negative perspectives of the pupil. This may very well be true, however, the adoption of this persona by a pupil is also a response to the marginalization and rejection that they experience through racism. In many respects, it might be seen as an attempt to establish their own identity – away from the whiteness that rejects them but in some respects they cannot escape from. In some ways, their need to adopt a black rebellious identity is almost a caricature of the culture they wish to identify with in order to overcome their own whiteness (Song 2003).

The contradictions of mixed-race realities

As mixed-race children struggle to create an identity and respond to the racism around them, the evidence suggests that they are also capable of being racist themselves. Tizard and Phoenix (2002) found that 53 per cent of their survey sample admitted to being racist at sometime or other. In terms of the sample, this meant that White/Black children targeted mainly Asian people, while whites were rarely the object of their racism. The following is a survey response from Tizard and Phoenix (2002):

> 'I've been jokedly racist, but then sometimes I've said it seriously, but luckily the person took it as a joke anyway. [Who have you said it to seriously to?] This kid X, like, all of us was mucking about, and we just kept slagging each other off and mouthing, and I just said, "Shut up you smelly Paki" ... Although I'd said it a couple of times before jokedly, that time I said it I meant it, sort of, but that's the only thing ever, I think.'

(154)

The above illustrates the tensions in the young people's lives in terms of their own ethnic and cultural identities: the contradictions they feel about their own ethnic and racial identity and how they should relate to other ethnic minority groups. In part, they recognize a need for solidarity yet at the same time there is distance from the notion of being a member of an ethnic minority group. It is a similar response to that of the Afro-Caribbean boys, who, in the 1970s, were members of gangs that were predominately white and used to go 'Paki-bashing'. This undertaking of clearly racist violence against another ethnic group was a denial of their position in society's ethnic and racial hierarchy. This process may be an attempt to overcome the alienation of self by adopting the language and attitudes of the more vocal racist white discourses against other minority groups. The child, by dint of circumstances, must choose their own racial identity, which is not an issue for their mono-racial peers (Herman 2004). The very process of choosing clearly imposes an emotional and psychological stress on the child (ibid.). The adoption of the white racist discourse in their relationships with other minority ethnic groups could be viewed as a response to their identity predicaments just as much as the adoption of a rebellious black persona by some children, as described above. It is in other words, the other side of the coin. Whatever perspective they adopt the central issue confronting many mixed-race individuals is frequently one of desiring acceptance and a need for belonging.

Parents of mixed-race children

The parents of mixed-race children have dilemmas at a number of different levels, including their own relationship with their partner and, of course, their relationship with and to their own children (Alibhai-Brown 2001). This latter concern is clearly demonstrated in the views of Lowri Turner (see the quote at the beginning of this chapter). That the parents face challenges in a racist society is not surprising. Alibhai-Brown (2001) quotes a powerful and emotionally charged description of the responses that individuals face in interracial relationships:

> 'I feel uneasy walking down the street with him, or taking public transport. There is a flicker of uneasiness in white men's eyes partly because black men with white women is one of the last great sexual taboos of our times. On the other hand at parties I have been ignored by black women. I am worried about our future children being the target of racism because it's not something I grew up experiencing which will make it harder for me to know how to help them.'
>
> Jo-Ann Goodwin, a freelance journalist, who is married to a Brazilian interviewed in the *Daily Mail* in 1996 (Alibhai-Brown 2001: 125)

The difficulties that couples face in their relationships do not just relate to a white/black relationship but also within the officially invisible mixed-race and ethnic partnerships. Alibhai-Brown (2001) also cites the experiences of a Sikh man, Gurinder, who fell in love with a Muslim woman in 1996; he recalls a violent experience as a reaction to his relationship:

> 'They burn my hands. See? They scarred my face with a sharp pen. They tried to get me to kill myself by sitting around me and giving me Panadols in my hand. Go, they said, die before you bring shame and marry a Muslim.'
>
> (125)

It should be noted in the case of Gurinder it was members of his own community that were committing this violence against him. The response to mixed-race or intercultural relationships can be extremely violent for the individuals concerned. The two main issues that bring forth this violent reaction are 'colour', in other words 'blackness' (see the quotes at the beginning of the chapter), and religion. Both these elements are part of the social cement that binds people together in their ethnic and cultural groups. To step outside is often regarded as unacceptable by the communities to which they belong. The social forces that individuals in mixed-race, interracial or inter-ethnic relationships confront place a great deal of strain on them as individuals and can adversely affect the relationship.

The children of a mixed-race relationship will be acutely aware of how their parents' relationship is viewed not only by the wider society, but often by the extended family to which they belong. Tizard and Phoenix (2002) identify that the most frequent form of discrimination that mixed-heritage young people are aware of is that practised by their parents' family. The Tizard and Phoenix (2002) study also found that even though a person may be in a mixed-race relationship, they could also still express and exhibit racist behaviours. For example, they cite one child as saying: 'My [white] mother does tend to blame blacks for quite a lot of things, she says a lot of the time they ask for it' (157).

Blaming and expressing negative views about the ethnic group from which one's partner comes from should not be a surprise, the rationale for such thought processes may be that 'All the stereotypes are true but I have married the exception'. Whatever the reasoning or lack of reasoning that goes into these attitudes, this does demonstrate the complexity of human relationships. As an example, the author once met a couple – a white male and black woman. The male partner was an active member of the far-right racist National Front. What needs to be recognized is that all couples face problems and dilemmas due to the nature of their relationship from social forces external to the relationship; this applies as much to mixed-race relationships as to mono-racial partnerships. The external socio-cultural and political forces also have an impact on the children produced by the relationship. It is not possible to escape the environment and the dominant ideas in the community and society in which the individual lives – resistance is always possible but ideas such as racism will still exist.

All parents of mixed-race children express a concern for their future well-being, however, in the Tizard and Phoenix (2002) study over half of the parents interviewed underestimated the level of racism that their children encountered both at school and in the community in general. The one area that parents are more often aware of is name-calling at primary school. What is evident is that the colour of the parent is crucial in understanding the experiences that their children might be going through. The black or ethnic minority parent is more aware of and sensitive to the problems that their child might encounter compared, if relevant, to the white parent. This seems an obvious conclusion, as a white person's experience of racism from the dominant community will only be through second-hand experiences through relationships and/or friends.

What is also important is the recognition of ethnicity and race adopted by the parents. The white parent will often encourage their mixed-race child to think of themselves as black. In part, this represents an understanding of the way their child will be perceived by the wider society, and, therefore, providing the child with the emotional and intellectual tools to deal with their coming experiences. However, it also represents a denial of their ethnicity and cultural heritage. Racism is creating, in some respects, a divide between the parent and the child. The children are not conceived as being the same, both by the parent and the wider community. To a certain degree, the child and parent suffer from an alienation from each other due to the gulf that is based on notions of race. The extent of and the form that this alienation takes will depend on the actual experiences that both parent and child will go through over time.

Student reflection

Think about the following question and attempt to justify your answer.

- Why shouldn't a mixed-race person who is part white and part Afro-Caribbean be thought of as white instead of black as they are currently?

Conclusion

The chapter has dealt with aspects of the social realties of individuals identified or self-identified as mixed-race. The difficulty in any discussion of mixed-race is the difficulty of definition. The problems do not stop with definition, for the very language used is problematical, not only in terms of its acceptability – clearly half-caste is racist, unpleasant and offensive. However, the very term used in this chapter, mixed-race, has been objected to (see above). The question then arises: What language, labels, terms should be used to describe someone who is the child of parents from different racial, ethnic and possibly cultural backgrounds. Do the alternative descriptors such as interracial and dual-heritage provide a more accurate portrayal? Do they provide a clearer picture of what is a highly charged issue, one more to do with ideologies of race than the realities of people? Once in the slave-owning societies of the Caribbean, individuals with what was termed 'one drop of black blood' were deemed to be black. These societies had specific terms to define individuals in a complete racial hierarchy based on the supposed amount of blackness within them: an octoroon was a person who was supposedly one-eighth black and a quadroon was a person one-quarter black – in both cases this suggests that an individual some generations back was supposedly black. The amazing reality is that the octoroon individual may have looked 'white', could even 'pass' as 'white' but in terms of slave-owning societies they were black but edging nearer to white. This represented a hierarchy of power based in part on race but also on the context of imperial power. Today, no one would use terms such as octoroon but their use in the past exposes the fallacy of race.

Race is a social construct that draws boundaries between the acceptable and the unacceptable. Race identifies the dominant socio-political discourse in society and justifies the subjugation of groups within a society. Racism is about power, privilege and access to resources. That race is, in some respects, an ambiguous boundary between people is demonstrated in the experience of Chinese people in South Africa, for during the apartheid era in South Africa, the Chinese community was given the status as honorary white. A mixed-race individual's very existence represents a challenge to these boundaries and the very notion of race and miscegenation. As indicated at the start of the chapter, it is not possible to discuss issues such as race without considering the socio-economic and political context of the time. The growth of a sizeable population of mixed-race individuals sits alongside the contradiction of the growth of racism in society generally. This will present even more challenges to the individual concerned for their very identity will become an issue, just as the national identity for Muslims living in the UK is presently an issue. Just as Muslims are almost deemed to be a religious fifth column and a threat to Western values and culture, the mixed-race individual may be represented in the same way.

Key points

- Race is a social construct and has no basis in biology.
- Mixed-race is a term that is linked to an individual's blackness rather than a descriptor of any genuine dual heritage.
- Any definition of mixed-race is problematic.
- Mixed-race individuals experience racism from a number of perspectives.
- Mixed-race parents do not always perceive their children as the same as themselves.
- The academic achievement of mixed-race individuals varies from group to group.
- Some mixed-race groups are officially invisible – they are not recognized in official statistics
- Any discussion of race must take into account the socio-political and economic conditions of the society that is under review.

Recommended reading

Fannon, F. (2008) *Black Skin, White Masks*, London: Pluto Press.
Fryer, P. (1984) *Staying Power: The History of Black People in Britain*, London: Pluto Press.
Olumide, J. (2002) *Raiding the Gene Pool: The Social Construction of Mixed Race*, London: Pluto Press.
Parker, D. and Song, M. (eds) (2001) *Rethinking Mixed Race*, London: Pluto Press.

References

Ali, T. (2002) *The Class of Fundamentalisms: Crusades, Jihads and Modernity*, London: Verso.
Alibhai-Brown, Y. (2001) *Mixed Feelings: The Complex Lives of Mixed-Race Britons*, London: Women's Press.
Aspinall, P. (2000) The challenges of measuring the ethno-cultural diversity of Britain in the new millennium, *Policy and Politics*, 28 (1): 109–18.
—— (2003) The conceptualization and categorization of mixed race/ethnicity in Britain and North America: identity options and the role of the state, *International Journal of Intercultural Relations*, 27: 269–96.
Asthana, A. and Smith, D. (2009) Revealed: the rise of mixed-race Britain, *Observer*, 18 January.
Bellos, L. (2007) I loathe the term 'mixed race' …, in J. M. Sims (ed.) *Mixed Heritage – Identity, Policy and Practice*, London: Runnymede Trust.
Caballero, C., Haynes, J. and Tikly, L. (2007) Researching mixed race in education: perceptions, policies and practices, *Race, Ethnicity and Education*, 10 (3): 345–62.
Fekete, L. (2009) *A Suitable Enemy: Racism, Migration and Islamophobia in Europe*, London: Pluto Press.
Gillborn, D. (2008) *Racism and Education: Coincidence or Conspiracy?* London: Routledge.
Gordon, L. (2004) Race, biraciality, and mixed race, in J. Ifekwunigwe (ed.) *Mixed Race Studies: A Reader*, London: Routledge.
Herman, M. (2004) Forced to choose: some determinants of racial identification, *Multiracial Adolescents in Child Development*, 75 (3): 730–48.
Kunonani, A. (2007) *The End of Tolerance: Racism in 21st Century Britain*, London: Pluto Press.
Montagu, A. (1997) *Man's Most Dangerous Myth: The Fallacy of Race*, 6th edn, New York: Altamira Press.
Owen, C. (2001) Mixed race in official statistics, in D. Parker and M. Song (eds) *Rethinking Mixed Race*, London: Pluto Press.
Platt, L. (2009) *Ethnicity and Family: Relationships within and between Ethnic Groups: An Analysis*

Using the Labour Force Survey, Essex: Institute for Social & Economic Research, University of Essex.

Runnymede Trust (1992) 'Race and Immigration: Runnymede Trust Bulletin' cited in Gillborn, D. (1995) *Racism and Antiracism in Real Schools: Theory, Policy, Practice*. Buckingham: Open University Press.

Song, M. (2003) *Choosing Ethnic Identity*, London: Polity Press.

—— (2007) The diversity of 'the' mixed race population in Britain, in J. M. Sims (ed.) *Mixed Heritage – Identity, Policy and Practice*, London: Runnymede Trust.

Tikly, L. (2007) Meeting the educational needs of mixed heritage pupils: challenges for policy and practice, in J. M. Sims (ed.) *Mixed Heritage – Identity, Policy and Practice*, London: Runnymede Trust.

Turner, L. (2007) 'I love my mixed race baby – but why does she feel so alien?', *Daily Mail*, 13 July.

Tizard, B. and Phoenix, A. (1995) The identity of mixed parentage adolescents, *Journal of Child Psychology and Psychiatry*, 36 (8): 1399–1410.

Tizard, B. and Phoenix, A. (2002) *Black, White or Mixed Race? Race and Racism in the Lives of Young People of Mixed Parentage*, revised edn, London: Routledge.

Part 2

The developing child

This part of the book explores three significant areas in relation to the development of the child – child psychology, child language development and child sexuality.

The first chapter in this part by Gallard explores the differing models of psychological development of children, alongside the key psychological approaches to childhood. The fact that psychology, as a science, seeks to utilize subjectivity when considering childhood is highlighted, as are the dangers of making assumptions about child development and, therefore, stereotyping children. Gallard highlights the necessity of taking a critical approach to the major psychological theories of child development in order to avoid this.

The main tenet of the discussion is the importance of dualism when considering the psychological development of children. Children do not develop and mature in a vacuum, that is, psychological development is interdependent on external influences. In other words, children's inner worlds are mediated by external influences within their environments, notably their peers and significant adults.

The importance of external input on child development is a major part of the discussion in Murphy's chapter on child language. This chapter outlines the milestones of typical child language development in light of the principal traditional theoretical approaches to child language development – the nature versus nurture debate. The chapter then goes on to consider the correlation between low socio-economic status and delayed language development, and the devastating consequences this can have on the literacy levels, educational achievement and overall life chances of the individual.

Murphy describes the current language development crisis which is occurring in the UK in which upwards of 60 per cent of children in some areas of social disadvantage are starting school with speech, language and communication needs. As research indicates that one of the major reasons for differing rates of language development between lower and higher socio-economic groups is the quantity of input they receive, Murphy suggests that the current situation may cause us to reconsider the nature versus nurture debate.

Clarke's chapter on childhood sexuality explores a topic which is rarely dealt with at length in books about childhood. For, as Clarke notes, in contemporary society the association of childhood and sex is taboo and controversial and the general conception is that children are, or should be, asexual. This, however, has not always been the case historically, and psychoanalysts such as Freud assert that children are, indeed, sexual beings. Clarke discusses the repression of child sexuality and its consequences, such as the high incidence of homophobic bullying in schools. He suggests that the repression and denial of children's sexuality is associated with social and political control and that it is impossible to separate arguments about sexuality from broader debates about the rights of children and the role of adult power in controlling their lives. Clarke concludes that in order to protect children's well-being and sexual health, and to ensure that their self-determination is reconciled with the prevention of abuse, rather than silence children on the subject of sex, adults should listen to their views and preferences and respond to their needs.

2.1   The psychology of the child
Mind games

Diahann Gallard

Psychology and childhood

The term 'psychology' brings together the Ancient Greek suffix meaning 'study' (*ology*) and the prefix meaning 'soul' (*psyche*), and it is generally defined as the 'science of the mind' (yet not to be confused with the same term used by Holmes (1921) for his idea of 'Religious Science'). Psychology is a science-based discipline which contributes to our understanding of how children develop and learn, alongside the other aligning disciplines, for example philosophy and sociology. Of the many psychology textbooks, most are filled with views and ideas formulated into theories to help understand elements of child development. But what does psychology really contribute to our knowledge of childhood? That question in particular is the focus of this chapter.

Childhood is viewed as a phase of development for humans between birth and adulthood which, in British culture, is 18 years of age. However, according to Moore (2001), the period of change can be viewed as elastic in length and tying in with the end of the phase that most people complete their education which, due to increasing numbers in higher education, could be viewed as 21. Thus, it is clear that there are complexities when attempting to focus on a specific age range. In fact, many theorists (Erik Erikson, Lawrence Kohlberg etc.) see no distinct childhood phase. Also, the field of 'developmental psychology' is often assumed to centre on the psychology of *childhood*, when in fact it is a scientific study of how we grow and develop (physically and mentally) throughout our lifespan from conception until death (Davenport 1988). As such, this chapter will consider the contributions of psychology to the childhood phase but also what psychology tells us about our *conceptions* of childhood.

Activity 2.1.1: The child at seven

Take a few moments and imagine a seven-year-old child.
  Now try to answer the following questions:

* What are the general features of the scene in your mind?
* Are you thinking about what the child looks like and acts like, or are you thinking about what they are doing?

If you are mostly focusing on what the child looks like and acts like then you would be interested more in how nature provides variation in 'traits' (attributes derived from our genetic makeup), but if you are focusing more on the activities that the child is taking part in then, perhaps, you would be mostly interested in how our experiences can shape who we are (a nurturist point of view). Regardless of your leaning of viewpoint in the 'nature versus nurture' debate, we do need to recognize that, seeing as humans are social beings (where we must exist alongside others from birth), the 'doing' part within the general scene is important.

Was your imagined child playing? This is an activity viewed by some psychologists as a means of making sense of the world or for knowledge and meaning construction (Piaget 1954). Where some psychologists differ is with the role that adults should assign themselves for this activity. Jean Piaget (1896–1980) believed that proximal-distance observation (with involvement only required for providing appropriate materials) was essential to allow children hands-on, experimental experiences for optimum meaning-making for the individual in the world in which they live. In contrast, Lev Vygotsky (1896–1934) saw ongoing and sustained sensitive intervention by adults as a means to allow children to gain shared and relevant understanding (with meaning) of their specific social world.

When considering the *doing* part of a childhood scene (often termed 'behaviour'), a psychological perspective can also contribute to how we view childhood behaviour. Going back to your imagined child in your response to Activity 2.1.1 – was your child 'good' or 'naughty' (or somewhere in between)? If their behaviour had negative elements you could view this as being due to either internal processes (for example, wilfulness or contrariness) or external dynamics (underachieving to the level of expected conformity to social norms and niceties imposed in their culture). What is important is that psychologists will tend to consider both. Dualism is an important concept in psychology as it distinguishes between our mental world and the physical world, although some theorists view these processes as interactive (separate but interacting, as viewed by Descartes (see Christofidou 2001)) or in parallel (together but in tandem, as viewed by Titchener (2005) [1915]).

Was your imagined child based on someone you have met in real life, or a pure creation of your imagination (i.e. a blend of assumed character 'traits')? This is an important point as it may indicate whether you recognize that scientific observation differs from *assumptions*. What social psychology tells us is that we often make judgements and stereotype people, which can be rational but inaccurate. What is happening when we make attributions for what we see and hear regarding others is our brain attempting to do the least cognitive work and expenditure of effort, where our brain is making shortcuts and using prior examples to construct 'a type' (Baron and Byrne 2003). If professionals working with children apply these stereotypes then the shadow effect of this is not then recognizing the *individuality* of the child. Further, when we stereotype children we are not taking account of what is happening in both the interior world and exterior world for that unique child, in their specific situation, for just that moment in time. A key psychological theorist has attempted to recognize this – Bronfenbrenner's Ecological Systems Theory (1977; 1979; 1989) provides a model for viewing children in this way (of seeing an individual in their cultural context at a precise point of a timeline).

Again returning to your imagined child from Activity 2.1.1, if you were able to construct your 'typical child' in your imagination (mind's eye) this indicates that you have already have a classified 'CHILD' as a general category (schema) and you are likely to match all other children to this. In opposition to the idea of stereotyping is the idea of 'normalizing', which is another key psychological principle. Psychologists use the idea as a means to identify a typical kind, or average, for general human behaviour within the population (or 'normal distribution' across the population). This is termed 'normal' ('typical' or 'average') and the further from this norm a person is the more 'abnormal' they are (although the preferred term is now 'atypical'). Although this approach does have some elements of stereotyping, it is helpful for comparison and contextualization of many child development themes (i.e. by recognizing what 'typical' development should be we can become aware of high achievement or, conversely, problem development or behaviour. It is useful, particularly for when the identified need requires accommodation or intervention. Psychologists will then look at deficits of internal need versus the external need and make suggestions for adaption where appropriate (i.e. change the child versus change the environment).

Activity 2.1.2: Different perspectives on the child

How do you view 'a child'? Do you believe that children are 'little adults' or 'adults-in-waiting' or do you believe that children are a completely separate entity whereby there is only a change when the adult version emerges?

To help recognize and refine your viewpoint, try to answer the following questions:

- As a child were you just an immature version of yourself? Have your knowledge and views simply expanded or grown over time?
- Or alternatively, did you see, think and act completely differently as a child? Did your knowledge and behaviour shift a little bit at a time and from encountering critical events?

To help you further still:

- Do you believe that that we are able to discard childhood like a snake discards its skin as we reach the end of our teenage years?
- Is it possible that some characteristics of childhood remain with us?
- Is there possible dualism, where some of us change our physical characteristics to look adult but yet retain some childlike thinking and/or behaviour patterns?
- Due to environmental factors, are some children forced to mature faster than those of the same chronological age and as a result view the world in a more adult way?
- What type of experiences could change your outlook on life? Could a critical event prematurely jolt us out of our childhood phase completely?

The above are not questions that necessarily have answers, but you will see that once you try to *think* of the answers, that specific definitions of childhood will differ depending on your individual viewpoints to the above and the experiences *you* have had. What would anyone who is *not you* say about childhood (i.e. the wider population)? Psychologists attempt to remove the subjectivity, and focus more on objectivity, when considering childhood. This is done either by seeking the views of everyone (or enough to be deemed representative of the population) or by providing conditions to repeatedly test the assumptions we have about childhood. This is why psychology is a science-based discipline.

By using a psychological perspective you also begin to look at a child not for *who* they are (i.e. genetic inheritance and birth) but *how* they are (of how we, although all human, come to be so individual and different to each other) and what they could be, or their 'individual potential'. Two main approaches to child development help us to do this. These are the 'biological approach' and the 'learning approach'.

The biological approach provides us with evidence and explanations as to whether our physical and mental characteristics are mainly dictated by our genetic make-up. Theorists such as Arnold Gesell and John Bowlby view our development as pre-set, with a gradual unfurling in response to key events in our childhood phase. As such our innate (set) traits are 'triggered' by experience, with the degree of the traits' expression moderated by certain experiences during our life course. 'Maturationist' theorists see this pathway as an incremental and sequential process that leads children from immaturity to adulthood, whereby individuals show maladaption and deviate from their optimum development if key experiences are delayed or omitted. However, the alternative perspective is via the learning approach which centres on our life context and experiences and aligns to John Locke's 'tabula rasa' (blank slate). This approach suggests that our post-birth physical development, knowledge construction and views of self are entirely due to the context of our lives.

At the start of the chapter you were asked to imagine a child. Now a child and a scenario will be provided for you.

Case study: Elliot

Elliot is six years old and the third child in a family of four. Elliot is described by his parents as being 'the hardest work' of their children. His mother and father both work full-time and are thus reliant on a strong family network of grandparents, aunties and uncles to help out with the children. As well as his siblings, Elliot has many cousins to play with on a regular basis. One day, Elliot pushes one of his same-age cousins down the stairs. Elliot's parents were present and are available to deal with the issue at once (the other child is slightly bruised but otherwise unharmed). They are angry with Elliot for his behaviour and let him know that his actions are unacceptable. They apologize to the child and the child's parents and they make a fuss of the hurt cousin, and Elliot is directed to apologize to the cousin and has to part with one of his toys temporarily as a 'punishment'. That evening the parents sit down and calmly discuss the event.

Why did Elliot behave that way? Why does Elliot often cause negative situations such as this? Can they do anything to pre-empt or prevent further negative behaviour?

- Firstly, what different reasons can you think of that explain Elliot's behaviour?
- How would using a psychological approach explain Elliot's behaviour?

The assumption quite often made with scenarios such as the above is that there is something wrong with Elliot or that his psychological processes have digressed from normal behaviour. We hold an image of a 'perfect child' in our mind and compare any behaviour we observe in children against this norm. In the case study of Elliot it is important to recognize the key theme of 'normal distribution' across the population (as discussed earlier). Elliot's parents have seemingly ranked their children and Elliot would seem to be further away from their child norm, and as a consequence they wish to change him. What Elliot's parents will need to recognize is that our negative behaviour is only a problem in the context of other people (i.e. potential and actual 'victims' for our 'crimes') and that our actions become the environmental influence for others. In actual fact, Elliot's behaviour must be addressed because of health, safety and welfare implications for the child that he pushed and because it may indeed be indicative of individual potential for future difficulties for others he will meet during childhood and through adulthood.

Returning again to the case example, Elliot's behaviour as a snapshot observation may be interpreted as his having an 'off' day. The consideration of prior incidents of similar behaviour may be attributional, yet this still cannot be overlooked. In addition, we make assumptions that negative child behaviour has roots in deviance. Elliot may have, in fact, lashed out due to lack of foresight and from not considering or recognizing the outcome of the push and the wider context of being at the top of a flight of stairs. Often children do not have 'forethought'. Piaget and Inhelder (1967) acknowledged that children are born egocentric and only begin to move their thinking to incorporate other people and objects by the end of the pre-operational stage (by approximately seven years of age). Other theorists (Meltzoff 1995; Baron-Cohen 1991) later described this theme as 'theory of mind'. Therefore Elliot may be so focused on his own needs and emotionality that he cannot pay due attention to predicting possible outcomes involving others (i.e. he has not yet achieved 'theory of mind'). The pre-theory of mind state in childhood is viewed as highly typical. Elliot may just be immature in this domain. However, his lower rate of social and emotional development is not true for his siblings who share both genetic material and family experiences. We cannot disregard the possibility that he may not achieve 'theory of mind' in the future either, which is characteristic of Asperger's syndrome and autism (Frith 1989, Baron-Cohen, *et al.* 1993). This would be an innate basis of Elliot's behaviour. We should also recognize that some children can be highly empathic and considerate of others from an early age. The early experiences of sharing social experiences and other siblings can teach you that there are others as well as yourself and that sometimes their needs are in front of your own (a learned basis of behaviour). This influence has not significantly impacted for Elliot even with his extended family context. Elliot has lots of others in his social sphere to develop a high level of social awareness and empathy but this has not yet appeared to have taken effect. To consider this further would be an assumption; instead evidence over the remainder of childhood would need to be sought.

Other theorists would offer a different explanation for Elliot's behaviour based on what could be a learned response for prior event outcomes due to the context of life. Elliot could, perhaps, be more likely to act in a negative way. Behaviourist theorists (for example, John Watson, Burrhus Frederic Skinner, Ivan Pavlov) saw behaviour being determined by attention, reinforcement and learning. Elliot may be acting in a certain way because such negative behaviour is actually being reinforced by the attention he gets (due, perhaps, to wishing to gain attention within his large family context where he is constantly competing with others). Over time he may have learned that, although it is a negative behaviour he presents, it is actually the attention from others that is primary and desirable to him, and that any negative behaviour he displays actually proves more effective in this respect than his positive behaviour does.

Another key psychological theory that needs to be considered in the context of the case study is Bowlby's idea of 'attachment' (1969; 1973; 1980; 1988) in infancy leading to juvenile delinquency. Following on from Lorenz's (1935) view of 'imprinting', Bowlby considered adaptive social and emotional development as requiring an available mother figure that is stable, warm and constant within a 'critical period' following the birth of a child. The child has an innate archetype in their psyche (Jung 1970 [1916]) for this but it needs a physical expression in the early years of life. If the behaviour from this mother figure is adequate to the archetype then the child will interpret this as unconditional positive regard and general social acceptance. The child would learn to trust this attachment using the mother as a 'secure base' and they would be more likely to then go on to have healthy social relationships and emotionality and form multiple attachments in later life. It is possible that some disruption occurred when Elliot was an infant whereby he may have retained some attachment issues and be insecure with his positive regard. Elliot could be displaying the externalization of this internal conflict with those around him as part of resulting low self-esteem construct.

Social learning theorists would view Elliot's scenario slightly differently, instead explaining his behaviour as due to the assimilation of model behaviour, or 'modelling' (things we have observed others held in higher esteem do) and that our own behaviour will emulate elements of what we have observed (Bandura 1977). Again, this is assumed as typical for children as part of their ongoing social development. Elliot may have simply assimilated the behaviour that he has observed in others (for example that the method for conflict resolution in his family or society that he has observed is getting angry and physical displays of this anger) but Elliot then performs this to a greater extent.

Finally, with regard to the case study, there must be a consideration of whether the origin of Elliot's behaviour is due solely to his intrinsic motivation as an individual. Intrinsic motivation is the idea that Elliot actually derives satisfaction and fulfilment from his negative actions. Intrinsic motivation includes self-generated internal effort and an interest in mastering new things, plus *perceived control* of own actions (Heider 1958; Bandura 1982; Deci and Ryan 1985). It is within this concept that there is a potential for a dichotomy, which could be the urge toward 'good' or 'evil'. Whereas theorists such as Rogers (1961) believed we had internal curiosity and drive to be creative or 'good', there is also the potential for a human to display an internal drive to cause harm (Sternberg 1999), which would be the opposite domain of 'evil'. Within humanistic and transpersonal psychology this dichotomy is a major theme. Although criticized by some psychologists as an inadequate course for the study of the human experience, there is the idea that children will have an innate drive and ethical code for being the best person they possibly can be (the 'human potential movement'), which is a positive and affirming perspective of childhood. Yet alongside this viewpoint, psychologists pay due attention to the possibility of the reverse, of a descending innate drive for self-destruction or toward the harming of others, and a bleak and negative view of childhood. For Elliot, a usage of the second prognosis will have great implications for his view of himself, the view of his parents and any of the other people around him, and opens him up to the possibility of a 'self-fulfilling prophecy' (a prediction that causes itself to be true).

Activity 2.1.3: Good versus evil

- Do you believe that children can be born as either 'good' or 'evil'?
- What would be the outlook for children with either label in early childhood?
- What do you see as the potential for change for children?

This chapter has considered a range of psychological theories in order to illustrate how psychology can be applied to our understanding of childhood. The main theme that has been presented is that children have an inner world mediated by their external influences, and the impact of this for us as observers (as theorists or practitioners) and for the consideration of specific child development and behaviour issues. What is important to note is that the general practice of psychologists involves seeking a sense of balance between individual needs and the needs of others (i.e. recognition of the need for a defence of individual freedom that is recognized as *dependent on the needs of that individual's social and cultural setting*). By incorporating a psychological viewpoint, there is also recognition of how a child has interdependence with their peers and adults, and equally, how the experiences a child has resulting from interactions with others can influence that child's thoughts and behaviour. A consideration of this dynamic approach contributes a great deal to helping us to understand children, more so than a consideration of a child as a unitary concept. Children do not grow and develop in a vacuum and rarely become older and reach maturity with no social input or other environmental influences. By using psychological methods we have a tool for developing our collective knowledge of childhood, and specifically for understanding some of the factors that help with or, alternatively, hinder children reaching their individual potential.

Student reflection

Consider the contribution that inner nature and external influences have on the development of a child's psyche.

- Which factor do you think has a more profound effect on shaping the individual?

Key points

- Psychology is a science-based discipline which contributes to our understanding of children alongside other areas such as philosophy and sociology.
- Psychologists attempt to remove subjectivity when considering childhood by either seeking the views of everyone (or enough representatives) or by providing conditions to repeatedly test the assumptions we have about childhood.
- Psychologists disagree as to whether the childhood phase ends at a specific age or develops across a lifespan.
- Dualism is an important psychological concept. It concerns the internal processes (mental world) and external dynamics (physical world) and the relationship between them.
- Social psychology warns of the dangers of making assumptions about children (stereotyping) without recognizing their individuality.
- *Normalizing* (considering the typical or average) is a key psychological concern as the further from this norm a person is the more 'atypical' they are. This approach does have some elements of stereotyping, but it is helpful for comparison and contextualization of many child development themes (e.g. high achievement, issues with development or behaviour etc.)
- Two key approaches to child development are the 'biological approach' (genetic or pre-set development) and the 'learning approach' (development is related to life context and experience-based).
- When interpreting childhood behaviour psychologists can draw upon a range of theoretical models including theory of mind, intrinsic motivation, self-fulfilling prophecy, attachment and modelling.

Recommended reading

Baron, R. A. and Byrne, D. (2003) *Social Psychology*, 10th edn, Boston: Pearson Educational, Inc.

Davenport, G. C. (1988) *An Introduction to Child Development*, London: Collins Educational.

Smith, P. K., Cowie, H. and Blades, M. (2003) *Understanding Children's Development*, 4th edn, Oxford: Blackwell Publishing.

References

Bandura, A. (1977) *Social Learning Theory*, New York: General Learning Press.

—— (1982) Self-efficacy mechanism in human agency, *American Psychologist*, 37, 122–47.

Baron, R. A. and Byrne, D. (2003) *Social Psychology*, 10th edn, Boston: Pearson Educational, Inc.

Baron-Cohen, S. (1991) Precursors to a theory of mind: understanding attention in others, in A. Whiten (ed.) *Natural Theories of Mind: Evolution, Development, and Simulation of Everyday Mind Reading*, pp. 233–51, Cambridge, MA: Basil Blackwell.

Baron-Cohen, S., Tager-Flusbert, H. and Cohen, D. J. (eds) (1993) *Understanding Other Minds: Perspectives from Autism*, New York: Oxford Press.

Bowlby, J. (1969) *Attachment and Loss, Vol. 1: Attachment*, New York: Basic Books.

—— (1973) *Attachment and Loss, Vol. 2: Separation*, New York: Basic Books.

—— (1980) *Attachment and Loss, Vol. 3: Loss, Sadness and Depression*, New York: Basic Books.

—— (1988) *A Secure Base: Parent-child Attachment and Healthy Human Development*, New York: Basic Books.

Bronfenbrenner, U. (1977) Toward an experimental ecology of human development, *American Psychologist*, 32, 513–30.

—— (1979) *The Ecology of Human Development*, Cambridge, MA: Harvard University Press.

—— (1989) Ecological systems theory, in R. Vasta (ed.) *Annals of Child Development, 6*, pp. 187–251, Greenwich, CT: JAI.

Christofidou, A. (2001) Descartes' dualism: correcting some misconceptions, *Journal of the History of Philosophy*, 39 (2), 215–38.

Davenport, G. C. (1988) *An Introduction to Child Development*, London: Collins Educational.

Deci, E. L. and Ryan, R. M. (1985) *Intrinsic Motivation and Self-determination in Human Behaviour*, New York: Plenum.

Frith, U. (1989) *Autism: Explaining the Enigma*, Worchester, UK: Billing and Sons Ltd.

Heider, F. (1958) *The Psychology of Interpersonal Relations*, New York: Wiley.

Holmes, E. S. ([1921], 1957). *Creative mind and success*. New York: Dodd, Mead and Company.

Jung, C. G. (1970) [1916] *Collected Works, Volume 10*, London: Routledge and Kegan Paul.

Lorenz, K. Z. (1935). Der Kumpan in der Umwelt des Vogels (The companion in the bird's world), *Journal fur Ornithologie*, 83, 137–213. (Abbreviated English translation published 1937 in *Auk*, 54, 245–73.)

Meltzoff, A. N. (1995) Understanding the intentions of others: re-enactment of intended acts by 18-month-old children, *Developmental Psychology*, 31, 838–50.

Moore, S. (2001) *Sociology Alive!*, 3rd edn, London: Nelson Thornes.

Piaget, J. (1954) *Construction of Reality in the Child*, New York: Basic Books.

Piaget, J. and Inhelder, B. (1967) *The Child's Conception of Space*, New York: W. W. Norton.

Rogers, C.R. (1961). *On Becoming a Person: A Therapist's View of Psychotherapy*. Boston: Houghton Mifflin.

Sternberg, R. J. (ed.) (1999) *Handbook of Creativity*, New York: Cambridge University Press.

Titchener, E. B. (2005) [1915] *A Beginner's Psychology*, Boston, MA: Adamant Media Corporation.

2.2 The development of speech and language

Inborn or bred?

Lisa Murphy

Nobody is taught language. In fact you can't prevent the child from learning it.
— Noam Chomsky (1994)

Current research would suggest that there is a crisis occurring at the moment in relation to the development of early language among children in the UK. It is estimated that approximately 66 per cent of children have speech, language and communication needs (SLCNs). Moreover, it has been noted that the highest incidence of SLCNs among infants and toddlers is located in areas of social disadvantage and within families of low socio-economic status (SES) (Bercow 2008; I CAN 2007).

Approximately 16 per cent of these children have a specific communication disability which may be permanent or temporary (Lindsey and Dockrell 2002). These communication disabilities may result from cognitive, physiological, psychological or anatomical issues and may be part of a more generalized condition. The children experiencing such SLCNs are likely to need specialist help in school and beyond and may require alternative means of communication. It is vital that policy and provision identifies and caters for the needs of these children, their families and their educators as early as possible, so that they are able to reach their potential educationally and socially (Bercow 2008). Indeed, as there is an identifiable cause of disability, there is no reason why these children should not receive the personalized support that they need as soon as the SLCN is detected.

It is suggested here that the current crisis has reached its crescendo due to the remaining 50 per cent or so of children with SLCNs for whose needs there is no specific, identifiable physical or cognitive cause. The high levels of children currently entering preschool and school in the UK with SLCNs would seem to refute the quotation from Chomsky cited above. It seems at present that certain factors are, indeed, prohibiting many children with no specific physical or cognitive issues from learning language. Despite the current government's claim that *Every Child Matters* (DfES 2003) in certain sectors of our population some of the nation's children are starting their educational career at a linguistic disadvantage.

Developmental milestones in typical child language development

Table 2.2.1 provides a brief overview of the stages or developmental milestones of child language acquisition and development[1] during the first three years. Obviously, as children develop at individual rates, the ages given are approximate, though the sequence of stages appears to be fixed and universal to some extent (Fromkin, *et al.* 2003: 352). Before turning to a summary of some of the major theories of child language development, let us consider some aspects of the process of language acquisition in terms of the nature versus nurture dichotomy and in terms of the role of parent/adult input.

Clearly language acquisition and development is far from over after three years. Indeed, as Crystal (1986: 151–9) points out, children at four and five years of age have yet to master some of the more difficult consonant sounds and consonant clusters and, as they attempt to sort out the grammatical rules of the language, they make frequent errors such as mixing constructions, e.g. *Four green sweets, how old as me!* and confusing pronouns and reference, e.g. *A boy hurt hisself on the wall and it was bleeding.* Nevertheless, as children around three years of age begin to use the connective *and*, this could be argued as the last period of dramatic linguistic change: 'If any age has to be called a linguistic milestone, it has to be this' (Crystal 1986: 143). Children are now able to produce compound sentences and once they are over this hurdle, other conjunctions and the ability to form complex sentences follow fast.

Vocal and non-vocal behaviour from infants at the pre-linguistic stage suggests that that they are born with an innate or inbuilt disposition to interact and communicate, principally through sound, unless there is some form of impairment. Research in which syllables such as [ba] and [pa] were played over loud speakers to sucking infants have recorded, through changes in sucking rates, the infant's ability to discriminate between the sounds (Eimas, *et al.* 1971). Furthermore, it has been found that babies can distinguish between sounds that adult speakers cannot, for example, Japanese babies can discriminate between [r] and [l] while adult speakers of Japanese are unable to perceive or articulate a different phoneme here. The evidence suggests that infants are born with the potential to perceive sounds which are phonetically possible in any language, that is, they are innately multilingual.

From a very early age, infants will direct adult attention via gesture – initially gaze and later pointing. Gaze, head movements and exchanges of facial expressions, accompanied or unaccompanied by vocalization, constitute interactions and are the foundations of socialization and later conversational interaction. Tomasello, *et al.* (2007) assert that pointing rests on a joint attentional frame and describe two types of infant pointing which correlate to two types of universal communicative acts: protoimperative points and protodeclarative points. The former, similar to commands, are used to get an adult to retrieve an object, the adult being the agent in this situation. The latter are used to direct the adult's attention to an object which is part of the child's experience – in this case the object is the agent used to get the adult's attention. They conclude that, as pointing is universal and is based on the co-operative principle and social interaction, it is the logical precursor to the human universal of language whether verbal or non-verbal.

During the babbling stage children begin to segment vocalizations and this is believed to be the precursor to recognizing word boundaries (Mattys, *et al.* 1999). Deaf and hearing impaired infants also babble which could suggest that language and the predisposition to segment units of meaning is an innate facet of the human mind and is not dependent on input. However, some researchers believe that the babbling of deaf infants is, in fact, an imitation of the vocal gestures in speakers (Boysson-Bardies 1999) which would support a nurture approach to language acquisition. Moreover, Petitto, *et al.* (2001) found that when the infants of deaf parents are exposed to sign language as their first language they 'babble' with their hands. This could be cited as evidence for the argument that

Table 2.2.1 Stages of typical child language development[1]

Stage	Typical age	Features
Biological noises	0–2 mths	Gulping, coughing etc. Crying – reflective and intentional. Beginning to control air flow through vocal apparatus. Vowel-like sounds [a]. Some variety in pitch.
Cooing	2–6 mths	Great variety of sounds – beginning to control vocal chords and tongue, repetition of sound strings [mmm]. Consonant-like sounds and gradually some CV-like sounds [ɡa], [ka] – though as yet not identifiable with a specific language. No order of production of sounds. Lips being used, blowing raspberries – imitation of adult mouth movements. Throaty laughs. Practice with vocal tract muscles.
Babbling	6–12 mths	Reduplication of CV patterns [dadada]. Gradually becoming more varied in sounds and consonant/vowel-like combinations [adu]. Avoidance of complex sounds and consonant clusters [sp]. Initially may consist of random sounds, but 95% of consonants used are the 12 most frequent in world's languages. Gradually comes to include only those sounds in target language. Beginning to segment via intonation. Imitation of adult intonation.
One-word holophrastic stage	9–18 mths	Recognizable single words. Open-class words (nouns and verbs) – around 60% with a naming function related to objects in environment. Rate of acquisition 10–20 words a month. Avoidance of sounds due to difficulty of articulation produces non-adult-like articulations. Overextension (e.g. *apple* used for all round fruit in a shop) and underextension (e.g. *dog* used only for family dog, *cat* used for other similar four-legged animals) of word meanings. Growing use of social expressions and interactions. Gesturing – pointing begins around 11 months.
Two-word stage	18–24 mths	Rhythmic two-word utterances – fixed word order depending on word class – recognizable grammar? Questions evidenced by intonation. Negatives introduced. Introduction of some pronouns – *it, she* and prepositions – *on, off.* Increased number of sounds, but difficult sounds and consonant clusters still avoided – [sk], [f], [w]. Words shortened, syllables reduplicated – *wowo* for *water* – and some initial and final sounds dropped – *be* for *bed*. On average 50 words produced by 18 months, but 200 understood – comprehension/production gap of about 4 months. Overgeneralization of grammatical inflections – *goed, leaved.*
Telegraphic stage/ Multi-word stage	24–30+ mths	Initially, strings of words characterized by lexical (content) words with many grammatical (functional) words left out – *Man kick ball hard*. A variety of statements, questions and commands – *Where mummy go?* Gradual expansion in use of grammatical words and inflections – *-ing, -ed, -n't.* More complex verbal forms – *Fish might have a swim.* Vocabulary spurt around 30 months – little overextension. Pronunciation closer to adult, though still idiosyncratic – some sounds still problematic – [w], [r], consonant sounds as in ju**d**ge, plea**s**ure, **th**in, tea**ch**er, [br], [ɡr], [fl].

1 Table adapted from Crystal 1986: 34–141

language development is based on imitation and nurture as the babbling in such cases is related to the input a child receives.

From the two-word stage onwards most linguists would agree that children's utterances are rule governed in line with their first or target language(s). At the two-word stage most of the words used by children are open class or lexical words, that is, nouns and verbs, words which have semantic content. Some grammatical words with semantic content are also used. Children at this stage in most cases follow the word order of their target language(s). English speaking infants use *subject verb (object)* order from an early age, e.g. *mummy go*; *kick ball* (Brown 1973). Moreover, bilingual children will use appropriate word order for each of the languages they are developing when speaking that language and they tend not to confuse the two. The suggestion here is that some knowledge about syntax is innate, even when two grammatical systems are being developed.

From the two-word stage onwards children overgeneralize grammatical rules. For example, it is very common to hear a child use words such as *goed* or *drinked* or *mans* or *sheeps*. It would appear in such cases that the child is familiar with the rule for making the past tense in English by adding the suffix /ed/ to the present form and for making plural nouns by adding the suffix /s/ to the singular form. However, it is evident that the child has not yet mastered the rules for irregular past tense or plural forms.

The fact that the utterances produced by a child may differ phonologically, syntactically and semantically from those of adult speakers of the same language does not mean that the child's utterances are random and non-rule governed, but rather the utterances reflect the patterns of the language at a particular stage of development.

Learning or acquisition: theoretical approaches to child language development

For many years linguists and psychologists concerned with child language acquisition have centred their debate around the traditional dichotomy in discussions about learning – the nature versus nurture debate. In fact, the actual naming of the process by which children develop language has come under discussion. As Lyon (1981) points out, the terms language learning and language acquisition are both loaded to a certain degree. *Learning* inevitably carries the implications associated with a process which involves imitation, reinforcement, problem solving and conditioning. On the other hand, if we adopt the term *acquisition*, the suggestion is that acquiring language is 'coming to have something that one did not previously have', as Lyons states: 'if language is innate it is not acquired: it grows or matures naturally' (Lyons 1981: 252).

This quotation from Lyons indicates which side of the language acquisition debate he favours, however, most linguists and psychologists today would assert that language development is a combination of both innate structures and environmental input.

It is not the intention here to expound in detail the many and diverse theories which seek to explain the *miracle* or *mystery* of child language acquisition and development (Whitehead 2007: 1), as this has been done eloquently elsewhere (cf. Fletcher and Garman 1997; Fromkin, *et al.* 2003; Cattell 2007). However, a brief outline of the principal approaches to child language development which are relevant to the subsequent discussion of the current language crisis will be given.

The crux of the debate about the mechanisms of child language acquisition and development revolves around a central dichotomy:

- Human language development is a form of behaviour and, like the behaviours of all living organisms, including human beings, is learned through a process of stimulus, response and reinforcement which modify and mould the behaviour, that is, through operant conditioning.
- The capacity to develop language is a unique human competence which is inbuilt or innate in the human mind and takes the form of a language acquisition device (LAD). The LAD, once it has been triggered by minimal and limited environmental input, uses this input, mostly unconsciously, to work out the rules or parameters of a specific language in relation to its embedded set of principles or universal grammar which can produce any possible human language.

The first theory was proposed by the American behavioural psychologist Skinner in his book *Verbal Behavior* (1957). Skinner had conducted experiments using rats and pigeons whose behaviour he modified through the process of operant conditioning. In this work he extended these findings to human behaviour, including language development. Another American academic, Chomsky, initially through a direct review of Skinner's work, 'A review of *Verbal Behavior* by B. F. Skinner' (1959), proposed the seeds of the second theory which was developed over time in his many subsequent works (1965; 1968 (2006); 1980; 2002).

Skinner's approach may seem plausible for a number of reasons, not least for the fact that we are all aware, from anecdotal experience, that children do imitate parents and other adults, linguistically and socially, and that much is learned via such imitation. Moreover, operant conditioning can be a very useful process for training individuals with language pathologies (Cattell 2007: 42). However, there are many factors in child language development which a behaviourist approach cannot explain adequately.

Firstly, as shown above, even at the pre-linguistic stage, infants, including hearing impaired infants, can perceive language and seem preconditioned to communicate via language. Moreover, the stages of language acquisition, outlined in Table 2.2.1, to a large extent appear to be universal, which suggests that all human children are biologically hard-wired to follow this process, just as they are to eat or walk.

Secondly, if language development were merely a process of imitating modelled examples, storing them and repeating them at the appropriate time, what Cattell (2007: 39) terms the 'human tape recorder' theory of acquisition, it would take thousands of years to learn a language. This, and the sheer complexity of the system that most children master without formal teaching 'so quickly, given the immaturity of their other cognitive abilities and the lack of formal tuition' (Messer 2000: 138), calls the operant conditioning approach into question. These factors favour the concept of the LAD by which 'a child interprets the incoming linguistic data through the analytic devices provided by Universal Grammar [the principles], and fixes the parameters of the system [the language] on the basis of the analyzed data, his linguistic experience' (Chomsky 2002: 16). In other words, the LAD allows a child to work out the rules so that she/he can use them to generate all possible utterances in the language.

Let us reconsider children's overgeneralized mistakes discussed above. Even if we allow the possibility that an adult may once in a while make such an error that a child might imitate, this would not account for the fact that producing overgeneralizations, such as *swimmed* and *mouses*, is a phase that many, if not most, children go through. As Bee and Boyd (2007: 228) point out, 'imitation alone can't explain all language acquisition because it cannot account for children's tendency to create words and expressions they have never heard'. Rather, it could be suggested that these errors reflect the workings of the LAD as the child figures out and practises the rules of his/her language.

In contradiction to the behaviourist approach based on feedback and reinforcement, research has found that not only are children often resistant to correction (Peccei 2006: 2), but in the majority of parent–child interactions, when the child is in the early stages of language development, parents do not in fact correct grammatical inaccuracies but only the semantics or truth of the utterances. Hart and Risley (2004: 198) found only one adult correction of child grammar in 1,300 hours of data. Moreover, Chomsky (1980) argued that, given the nature of input children receive which is frequently grammatically inaccurate, incomplete, unstructured, full of hesitations and false starts, and noisy – what he termed *poverty of stimulus* – it would be impossible for them to develop accurate grammar by imitation.

Activity 2.2.1: Language development: nature or nurture?

- Having read the discussion above, summarize the evidence from research which supports either the nurture or nature side of the child language development debate. Which of the theories do you favour?
- Read Cattell (2007) chapter 15: explain what is meant by brain 'modules' and 'domains' in terms of language development.

Child-directed speech and nature versus nurture

Much research into child language development from the 1970s onwards focused on the input that children receive – possibly in response to Chomsky's *poverty of stimulus* claim. The fact that many adults change register when addressing children is common knowledge. Researchers such as Snow (1972), Ferguson (1977) and Sachs, *et al.* (1976) set out to define this parental input, or child-directed speech (CDS), and to assess its effects on child language development. Descriptions and discussions of the characteristics of CDS can be found elsewhere (see references above), but it is usually considered to be a simplified register of adult speech with reduced vocabulary, simplified and short sentence structures and special features of pronunciation such as a high pitch, over-articulation and a slow pace. During CDS exchanges adults are described as frequently repeating structures and recasting and expanding children's utterances in keeping with the syntactic accuracy of the target language.

Snow (1972) carried out research in which the interactions between mothers and children of varying ages were observed. She noted that the language of the adults was a more complex when speaking to older children than infants and she concluded that CDS, far from being a poor stimulus for children learning a language, is 'quite well designed as a set of "language lessons"' (ibid.: 561). Furthermore, she implied that due to this there was no need to attribute language acquisition to innate facilities.

Obviously, such bold claims were followed by counter-research. In sum, this research concluded that CDS is certainly a register of adult speech which is widely used by adults when interacting with infants, and which may, indeed, help infants to acquire their first language(s). However, there is no evidence to support the claim that it is fine-tuned to the infant's language capabilities; that it is an effective teaching tool; or that its use as a teaching tool refutes Chomsky's claim that language development is an innate human capacity

(Newport, *et al.* 1977, Shatz 1982). Further criticism of the work exploring CDS was that it was focused on parent–child interaction of a particular population – white, middle-class, Western families, in the majority of cases American, which might not be representative of the interactions experienced by all children (Hoff-Ginsberg 1991). Cross-cultural studies, such as Ochs and Schieffelin (1995), suggest that some cultures do not use a similar form of CDS with their young and, therefore, its use as a learning tool must be questioned.

Snow (1997: 72–3), in what Cattell (2007: 120) amusingly termed 'A Snow Drift', reconsidered her position in two *oversimplifications* (her terminology). The first point she conceded was that CDS is not necessarily the result of a conscious effort by mothers to teach their children to talk: 'most of the time they are simply trying to communicate with their children' and the modifications which constitute the features of CDS are a 'side effect' of this. Secondly, she stated that it was a misinterpretation of her findings to claim that there was no innate part of language ability. She wrote that it is 'absurd to argue' that any complex behaviour such as language is 'entirely innate or entirely learned' but it is not 'absurd to ask what proportion of the developmental variation ... is attributable to innate as opposed environmental factors'. Snow goes on to consider her own and Chomsky's stance on the relative importance of the two factors to effective language development. She states that:

> The prediction was made that children without access to such a simplified, redundant corpus [i.e. to CDS] would be unsuccessful or retarded in learning language. If such could be proven to be the case, then it could indeed be concluded that an innate, species-specific, linguistic component was relatively less important than Chomsky had hypothesized.
>
> (Snow 1997: 73)

In our discussion of the contemporary UK language crisis below we shall consider how the quantity and quality of input children receive is correlated to their language development, or, more worryingly their language delay, and what this correlation can tell us about the relative importance of input versus innate language faculties.

The current language crisis and its potential consequences

As mentioned above, it has been estimated that in some parts of the UK today, notably those areas of social disadvantage, upwards of 50 per cent of children are entering school or preschool with a primary SLCN for which there is no physical or cognitive cause (I CAN 2007; Bercow 2008). As communication is 'a fundamental human right' listed as one of the ten core life skills by the World Health Organization (Bercow 2008: 16), it is vital to the social, mental, educational and economic well-being of an individual.

There are a multitude of knock-on consequences of SLCNs which interfere with a person's life chances, particularly if the need is not identified and intervention is not put in place in the early years. Snowling, *et al.* (2001) report on a longitudinal study in which children with SLCNs whose needs were identified, supported and resolved by the time they were five years and six months were able to develop competent literacy skills and to follow a normal trajectory of attainment throughout their school career, finishing statutory education with comparable examination attainments as children who had had no previous SLCN. Unfortunately, early identification, intervention and resolution of SCLNs does not always occur.

There is not the space here to explore in detail the consequences that unresolved SLCNs may have on a person's life chances, such as bullying, social exclusion, failure to engage with the school curriculum, poor educational attainment, development of behavioural and emotional difficulties, poor employment prospects or long-term unemployment, mental health issues, low self-esteem, descent into criminality and drug abuse (cf. Bercow 2008; I CAN 2007). However, it is interesting to note some shocking statistics. Data from the National Pupil Database (cited in Bercow 2008: 18) shows that there is a huge difference in the numbers of children, with or without SLCNs, who achieve the expected levels in Standard Attainment Tests (SATs) at the end of primary school. There is a 55 per cent gap between the two groups for English, a 46 per cent gap for mathematics and a 41 per cent gap for science. When these children finish full-time statutory education, this difference in attainment remains roughly the same, with 15 per cent of young people with SLCNs attaining 5 GCSEs at A* to C, in comparison with the national average of 57 per cent.

Research has suggested that there is a very high incidence of SLCNs, between 55 and 100 per cent, among children with behavioural, emotional and social difficulties. Moreover, it has been estimated that of the 7,000 young people under 18 who pass through young offenders' institutions each year at least 60 per cent have a SLCN (Bryan 2004 cited in Bercow 2008: 41) and 50 per cent of the prison population in the UK are identified as having SLCNs in comparison to 17 per cent of the adult population overall (Basic Skills Agency 1994). It appears that adults with poor basic skills, including SLCNs, are less likely to co-habitate or marry, but when they do they are more likely to marry younger and have more children than average. This, coupled with poor employment prospects, suggests that adults with poor basic skills often live in social disadvantage, with low incomes, poor health, poor material circumstances, low self-esteem and limited motivation to improve their situation (Bynner and Parsons 1997).

Parent–child interaction: facilitating effective language development

Many studies (Hoff-Ginsberg 1991; Hart and Risley 2004; and references above describing CDS) have found that the following features of parent–child interaction are positive indicators of child language acquisition and development:

- engagement and joint attention – parent–child focus on same object, activity or event;
- response to child's chosen topic – casual and unplanned utterances;
- amount of talk;
- variety in topic and in vocabulary items used;
- length of utterances – despite earlier claims concerning CDS it has frequently been found that longer parental utterances have a positive impact on child language development;
- use of declaratives and questions, to elicit and maintain conversation;
- lack of directives (command) or prohibitions;
- variety in intonation and pitch patterns;
- imitation, recasting and expansion as child begins to engage in two or more word utterances.

As stated above, the current crisis in child language acquisition in the UK highlights a link between socio-economic status (SES) and SLCNs. In fact, the correlation between SLCNs, overall educational underachievement and social disadvantage is well documented. For decades research evidence, in the UK and USA, has suggested that academic underachievement of children from low-SES backgrounds can be directly related to language delay and low levels of language competence (Bernstein 1960, 1973; Labov [1969] (1970); Hart and Risley [1999] (2004), Ginsborg (2006: 10) refers to a survey carried out by Peers, Lloyd and Foster (2000) which suggested that UK children from low-SES backgrounds are nearly twice as likely to experience language delays than those from mid- and high-SES backgrounds, and that moderate and severe language delay is five times more likely in children from low-SES backgrounds. The obvious implication here is that parent–child interaction or CDS differs between the social classes and that the CDS of low-SES parents contains less of the positive indicators for child language development outlined above.

Research has found that this is indeed the case. Hart and Risley (2004) conducted a longitudinal observational study of the interactions between parents and children from three socio-economic backgrounds: professional, working-class and unemployed (on social welfare or benefits). They found that the interactions of parents from professional backgrounds displayed far more of the positive indicators for child language development than that of the other two groups. In fact, it could be suggested that the language of the professional group of parents in interactions with their child fitted the definition of CDS (see above) more than that of the others. This group of parents used an average of 30 affirmative comments per hour whereas the working-class group used an average of 15 and the unemployed group used an average of six affirmative, supportive comments per hour. The professional parents were more likely to offer guidance through questions rather than commands, to use language which focused on context-specific objects, events and relationships in order to keep the conversation going and they varied their talk and vocabulary more than the other groups. The most notable finding from this research, however, was the variation in time spent engaging with children between the parental groups and the sheer volume of talk that the parents used in their interactions: on average per hour the unemployed parents used 600 words, the working-class parents used 1,200 words and the professional parents used 2,100 words. Although they note the impact that quality of input has on child language development, Hart and Risley (2004: 193) state that 'the most important aspect of parent talk it its amount'.

This research was supported by that of Hoff-Ginsberg (1991) who analysed the talk of CDS of 30 low-SES mothers and 33 high-SES mothers in their homes in four different contexts: book reading, toy playing, mealtimes and dressing. In addition, the study explored the mothers' expectations of their children's language development and role as a conversational partner. Surprisingly, it was found that there were no significant differences in the mothers' expectations and attitudes towards their children's language development across the two groups. However, the expected differences in the CDS of the two groups were recorded in terms of richness of vocabulary, syntactic complexity, use of directives and affirmatives, and mother talk as contingent on children's, that is, eliciting conversation, responding to and continuing the child's topics.

The impact of each form of CDS on child language development has been borne out in numerous other studies (cf. Ginsborg 2006). In a nutshell, the CDS of higher-SES parents in general displays more of the positive indicators for child language development outlined above than that of low-SES parents. The fact that children from low-SES backgrounds are more likely to experience primary SLCNs and subsequent educational and social issues seems to suggest that one of the major contributing factors to child SLCNs is the CDS utilized by low-SES parents.

Activity 2.2.2: SES and language development

- What do you think could be the factors associated with low-SES which could affect child language development?
- Do you think that attributing delay in speech and language development to differences in CDS between low-SES and high-SES families is describing the language of low-SES families as deficient (cf. Ginsborg 2006: 17–22)?

Differences in CDS between socio-economic groups: possible causes

Research has suggested that, due to 'the oppressive effects of economic deprivation and environmental stress on human interaction' (Hoff-Ginsberg 1991:794), low-SES parents traditionally and typically spend more time in caretaking contexts, such as feeding and dressing, with their children and have less time and energy to engage in more leisure-based interactions such as book reading and toy play. Thus, it is in part the nature of the contexts that account for the differences in CDS: the caretaking context requires more directive and authoritarian parenting, and less free, unplanned and general talk. It was assumed that habitual engagement in a restricted set of caretaker contexts defines the nature of subsequent parent–child interactions in low-SES families. However, Hoff-Ginsberg's (1991) research found this not to be the case. It was expected that differences in CDS based on SES would be minimized in caretaker activities but more pronounced in the activities of book reading and toy play. Hoff-Ginsberg (1991: 793) found the opposite to be true. Although it was found that the pattern of intercorrelation between SES, CDS and context was somewhat complex, the difference between the groups was minimized in the more leisure-based activities and wider in the caretaking activities.

Oxford and Spieker (2006) conducted a longitudinal study examining how a set of risk indicators affected the preschool language development of 154 children of adolescent mothers. The researchers outlined six risk factors which from previous research were considered to have a negative impact on child language development: maternal verbal ability; maternal contextual risk, in terms of age, level of education, dependence on state welfare; home environmental risk in terms of language resources, such as age-appropriate books and toys; intergenerational risk in relation to level of grandmother's education and dependence of grandparents on welfare; relational risk measured by levels of secure or insecure attachment of child to mother; and the child's characteristics in relation to gender. The results of the research indicate clearly that the highest risk factors for normal child language development are poor quality home linguistic environment and maternal low verbal ability. Interestingly, poor home linguistic environment did not adversely affect language development when mothers had average or above verbal ability (ibid.: 167).

It would appear that differences in the nature of CDS within different SES groups are related directly to the verbal ability of the parent. Indeed, the study by Hoff-Ginsberg (1991) cited above revealed that the speech of low-SES mothers was different to that of high-SES mothers on two counts. In the first instance, in parent–child interaction it displayed fewer of the positive indicators of child language development given above. Moreover, in adult-to-adult interactions the speech of low-SES mothers contained overall fewer utterances, shorter utterances and less rich vocabulary than that of high-SES mothers. In other words, there was more difference between parent–child and adult-to-adult interaction within the high-SES group than in the low-SES group.

The evidence undeniably indicates that there are clear differences between the CDS of low-SES parents and of high-SES parents, that these differences are related to the language use of the parents in adult-to-adult interaction and that these differences have a direct effect on the language development of their children. This does not, however, advocate a deficit model of the language of low-SES adults, but suggests that such speakers are using a different code than high-SES speakers (Bernstein 1973). Furthermore, the evidence overwhelmingly suggests that one of the biggest differences between the CDS of different socio-economic groups relates to the volume of input from parents in terms of words per hour and length of utterance (Hoff-Ginsberg 1991; Hart and Risley 2004; Ginsborg 2006).

If we were to apply Chomsky's (1980) definition of *poverty of stimulus* to CDS, we could suggest that as all CDS is full of the hesitations, false starts, grammatical inaccuracies, the real poverty of stimulus is therefore no stimulus. As Hart and Risley (2004) state, though the quality of CDS is important for positive impact on child language development, the most important factor is ultimately the quantity of the input.

Current situation and lack of input

The crisis in early language development in the UK seems to be very much one of poverty of stimulus in terms of quantity of parental input. Research suggests that parents are confused about the process of child language development, do not realize the vital role that language input plays in child language development and do not understand reasons for SLCNs. Moreover, parents often fail to recognize the active role they have to play in child language development and often take language development for granted (Glogowska and Campbell 2004).

It could be argued that certain facets of contemporary lifestyles impede interaction between parents and children. Mealtimes have repeatedly been cited as an arena for positive family interaction and enhanced achievement of developmental milestones such as language development (Fiese and Schwartz 2008). However, there has been a steady decline in the UK and USA of families, particularly low-SES families, sharing communication-rich meals due to job strains and also due to the isolating effect of the media, for example. Forty-six per cent of families reported eating with the television switched on (Fiese and Schwartz 2008:7).

The effects of viewing television, including DVDs and other such media, on child language development have been well documented (see Close 2004 for a review of the literature), while the benefits of viewing age-appropriate programmes are acknowledged, excessive viewing is considered to have a detrimental effect on language development in all children, particularly those under two years of age. Moreover, it is regularly acknowledged that viewing television can benefit children's language development when interpreted through adult involvement. Unfortunately, with the high proportions of children who view television alone, often in their bedrooms, this is not always the case (Close 2004).

Zeedyk (2008), in collaboration with the 'Talk to Your Baby' campaign of the National

Literacy Trust, carried out research which found that children in the UK from birth to two-plus years spend on average two hours a day being transported in baby-buggies. The most frequently used buggy type is the away-facing buggy with 62 per cent of children observed in the study being transported in this way in comparison to 13 per cent being transported in towards-facing buggies. However, this wide-scale observation of parent–child interactions across a large number of cities in the UK found that parents were more than twice as likely to interact verbally with their children if they were in towards-facing buggies and that the behaviour of the parents predicted that of the children. Zeedyk (2008: 25–8) claims that this research may have far-reaching implications for parents, buggy manufacturers and the government. It is notable that towards-facing buggies are far more expensive than away-facing ones. Perhaps the interaction children are receiving in buggies is related to SES. Citing Hart and Risley (2004: 192), Zeedyk states that by the age of three the trajectories of children's communication and educational abilities are in place and this is affected by the linguistic interactions they have with parents. However, this is precisely the period of time, when a child's basic vocabulary is being put in place, that it receives least interaction from its parents in buggy rides.

In conclusion, it could be suggested that the crisis of early language development in the UK is occurring due to poverty of stimulus, but poverty of stimulus in terms of the amount of interaction between parents/adults and children. Snow's (1997) consideration of the Chomskyian principle of innateness versus input discussed above implies that, without access to appropriate CDS, children's language development will be restricted, which will evidence the fact that input is perhaps more important than innateness. Given the contemporary situation it would appear that Snow's contention is correct. The correlation between SLCNs and low-SES would suggest that mass education in terms of the importance of nurture and parental input on child language development is necessary within certain sectors of the population.

It is pleasing to note that the importance of speaking and listening as one of the bedrocks to future educational, social and mental well-being has not gone unnoticed by the government. As Bercow (2008) and I CAN (2007) point out, the importance of nurturing usual or normal language development and the necessity of early recognition and support for need, are central to many early years policies and initiatives, governmental and otherwise, such as, to name but a few: *Every Child Matters*, *Birth to Three Matters*, the Early Years Foundation Stage, Sure Start programmes, the Department of Health's Child Health Promotion Programme, the National Literacy Trust's 'Talk to Your Baby' campaign and the Basic Skills Agency's 'Talk to Me Project'. Notably, all of these initiatives stress the importance of quantity of talk and interaction between adult and child.

Student reflection

Reconsider the nature versus nurture debate about child language acquisition and development.

- Having read this chapter, what are your thoughts on this?

Key points

- Currently around 50 per cent of children in the UK have a SLCN for which there is no definable cause.
- Research has found that children from low-SES backgrounds are more likely to have a SLCN than others.
- Children who enter school with SLCNs are at a disadvantage socially and educationally and this can continue throughout life.
- Traditionally, theory concerned with explaining child language development has focused around the nature versus nurture dichotomy.
- Most linguists today believe that both nature and nurture are necessary for language development, however, the relative contribution of each is frequently debated.
- There are many features of CDS which seem to be positive indicators of child language development, most notably the quantity of input.
- Research has demonstrated a difference in CDS of low-SES and high-SES families, often in terms of the quantity of input.
- This may suggest that nurture, in the form of CDS, is the most important factor in effective language development.
- It would appear that certain sectors of the population need to be educated concerning the importance of parent–child interaction in the early years – indeed there are many initiatives which are at present attempting to address this.

Note

1 The terms *child language acquisition* and *child language development* are used interchangeably throughout this chapter. This is intentional due to the fact that the author perceives the process as a continuum. Moreover, the resistance to consistently insist on the term child language acquisition is somewhat influenced by the insightful analysis of the term provided by Lyons (1981: 252) – see page 52.

Recommended reading

Cattell, R. (2007) *Children's Language: Consensus and Controversy*, London: Continuum International Publishing Group Ltd.
Clegg, J. and Ginsborg, J. (eds) (2006) *Language and Social Disadvantage*, London: John Wiley & Sons Ltd.
Peccei, J. (2006) *Child Language: A Resource Book for Students*, London: Routledge.

References

Basic Skills Agency in Prisons (1994) *Assessing the Needs*, London: Basic Skills Agency.
Bee, H. and Boyd, D. (2007) *The Developing Child*, 11th edn, London: Allyn and Bacon.
Bercow, J. (2008) *The Bercow Report: A Review of Services for Children and Young People (0–19) with Speech, Language and Communication Needs*, London: Department for Children, Schools and Families (DCSF).
Bernstein, B. (1960) Language and social class: a research note, *British Journal of Sociology*, 11 (3): 271–6.
—— (1973) *Class, Codes and Control Volume 1*, London: Routledge and Kegan Paul.
Boysson-Bardies, B. de (1999) *How Language Comes to Children: From Birth to Two Years*, Cambridge, MA: Massachusetts Institute of Technology Press.

Brown, R. (1973) *First Language: The Early Stages*, London: Allen & Unwin.

Bynner, J. and Parsons, S. (1997) *It Doesn't Get Any Better: The Impact of Poor Basic Skills on the Lives of 37 Year Olds*, London: Basic Skills Agency.

Cattell, R. (2007) *Children's Language: Consensus and Controversy*, London: Continuum International Publishing Ltd.

Chomsky, N. (1959) A review of *Verbal Behavior* by B. F. Skinner, *Language*, 35: 26–58.

—— (1965) *Aspects of the Theory of Syntax*, Cambridge, MA: Massachusetts Institute of Technology Press.

—— [1968] (2006) *Language and Mind*, 3rd edn, Cambridge: Cambridge University Press.

—— (1980) *Rules and Representations*, Oxford: Basil Blackwell.

—— (1994) *The Human Language Series 2*, dir. Gene Searchinger, New York: Equinox Films/Ways of Knowing, Inc.

—— (2002) *On Nature and Language*, Cambridge: Cambridge University Press.

Close, R. (2004) Television and language development in the early years: a literature review. Available online at: http://www.literacytrust.org.uk/research/TV.pdf (accessed 22 April 2009).

Crystal, D. (1986) *Listen to Your Child: A Parent's Guide to Children's Language*, London: Penguin Books.

Department of Education and Skills (DfES) (2003) *Every Child Matters*, London: DfES.

Eimas, P., Siqueland, E., Jusczyk, P. and Vigorito, J. (1971) Speech perception in infants, *Science* 171: 303–6.

Ferguson, C. A. (1977) Baby talk as a simplified register, in C. Snow and C. A. Ferguson (eds) *Talking to Children*, Cambridge: Cambridge University Press.

Fiese, H. and Schwartz, M. (2008) Reclaiming the family table: mealtimes and child health and wellbeing, *Social Policy Report*, 22(4): 1–19. Available online at: http://www.sred.org/spr.html (accessed 22 April 2009).

Fletcher, P. and Garman, M. (eds) (1997) *Language Acquisition*, 2nd edn, Cambridge: Cambridge University Press.

Fletcher, P. and MacWhinney, B. (eds) (1995) *Handbook of Child Language*, Oxford: Blackwell.

Fromkin, V., Rodman, R., and Hyman, N. (2003) *An Introduction to Language*, 7th edn, Boston, MA: Thomson Wadsworth.

Ginsborg, J. (2006) The effects of socio-economic status on children's language acquisition and use, in J. Clegg and J. Ginsborg (eds) *Language and Social Disadvantage*, London: John Wiley & Sons Ltd.

Glogowska, M. and Campbell, R. (2004) Parental views of surveillance for early speech and language difficulties, *Children and Society*, 18: 266–77.

Hart, B. and Risley, T. R. [1999] (2004) *The Social World of Children Learning to Talk*, Baltimore, Maryland: Paul H. Brookes Publishing Co.

Hoff-Ginsberg, E. (1991) Mother-child conversations in different social classes and communicative settings, *Child Development*, 62: 782–96.

I CAN (2007) *The Cost to the Nation of Children's Poor Communication*, I CAN Talk Series 2. Available online at: http://www.ican.org.uk/sitecore/content/Home/Information//~Publications/cost tonationpdf.ashx (accessed 22 April 2009).

Labov, W. [1969] (1970) The logic of non-standard English, in F. Williams (ed.) *Language and Poverty: Perspectives on a Theme*, Chicago: Markham.

Lindsay, G. and Dockrell, J. (2002) *Educational Provision for Children with Specific Speech and Language Difficulties in England and Wales*, London: Cedar and the Institute of Education, University of London.

Lyons, J. (1981) *Language and Linguistics*, Cambridge: Cambridge University Press.

Mattys, S. L., Jusczyk, P. W., Luch, P. A. and Morgan, J. L. (1999) Phonotactic and prosodic effects on word segmentation in infants, *Cognitive Psychology*, 38: 465–94.

Messer, D. (2000) State of the art: language acquisition, *The Psychologist*, 13 (3): 138–43.

Newport, E., Gleitman, L. and Gleitman, H. (1977) Mother, I'd rather do it myself: some effects and non-effects of maternal speech style, in C. Snow and C. A. Ferguson (eds) *Talking to Children: Language Input and Acquisition*, Cambridge: Cambridge University Press.

Ochs, E. and Schieffelin, B. (1995) The impact of language socialization on grammatical development, in P. Fletcher and B. MacWhinney (eds) *Handbook of Child Language*, Oxford: Blackwell.

Oxford, M. and Spieker, S. (2006) Preschool language development among children of adolescent mother, *Applied Developmental Psychology*, 27: 165–82.

Peccei, J. (2006) *Child Language: A Resource Book for Students*, London: Routledge.

Petitto, L., Holowka, S., Sergio, L. and Ostry, D. (2001) Language rhythms in baby hand movements, *Nature*, 413: 35–6.

Sachs, J., Brown, R. and Salerno, R. (1976) Adult's speech to children, in W. von Raffler Engle and Y. Lebrun (eds) *Baby Talk and Infant Speech*, Lisse: Peter de Ridder Press.

Shatz, M. (1982) On mechanisms of language acquisition: can features of the communicative environment account for development?, in E. Wanner and L. Gleitman (eds) *Language Acquisition: The State of the Art*, Cambridge: Cambridge University Press.

Skinner, B. F. (1957) *Verbal Behavior*, Englewood Cliffs: Prentice-Hall.

Snow, C. (1972) Mothers' speech to children learning language, *Child Development*, 43: 549–65.

—— (1997) Conversations with children, in P. Fletcher and M. Garman (eds) *Language Acquisition*, Cambridge: Cambridge University Press.

Snow, C.E. and Ferguson, C.A. (eds) (1977) *Talking to Children*, Cambridge: Cambridge University Press.

Snowling, M. J., Adams, J. W., Bishop, D. V. M. and Stothard, S. E. (2001) Educational attainments of school leavers with a pre-school history of speech-language impairments, *International Journal of Language and Communication Disorders*, 36 (2): 173–83.

Tomasello, M., Carpenter, M. and Lizkowski, U. (2007) A new look at infant pointing, *Child Development*, 78 (3): 705–22.

Whitehead, M. (2007) *Developing Language and Literacy with Young Children*, 3rd edn, London: Paul Chapman Publishing.

Zeedyk, S. (2008) *What's Life in a Baby Buggy Like? The Impact of Buggy Orientation on Parent-Infant Interaction and Infant Stress*. Available online at: http://www.literacytrust.org.uk/talktoyourbaby/pushchairs_research.html (accessed 22 April 2009).

2.3   Childhood sexuality
Coming of age

John Clarke

Books about childhood seldom deal with issues of sexuality at any length. The reasons for this are obvious. In themselves, sex and sexuality are topics that excite embarrassment and controversy for most people whatever society they live in. Despite the prevalence of sex and sexually related material in much of the popular media, there remain taboos and social limits placed on discussing or describing sex in public and in private. When we deal with sex in any setting, we raise issues which go beyond the biological processes involved. Sex is concerned with power and the way different people exert power over others in their relationships. It is deeply implicated in issues of morality and deeply held views of how we should live. Indeed for some people morality and acceptable sexual behaviour are virtually synonymous. How often do we hear people who condemn gay relationships or teenage promiscuity with a passion that they are unable to display when talking about cruelty or avarice? Sex makes a link between our personal lives and the social relationships we enter into. It is intimately related to gender and gender differences and our personal models of what gender identity means. In religious terms sex is closely tied up with issues of sin, guilt and innocence. Unsurprisingly this has always been an area fraught with difficulty and anxiety. When there is any attempt to link sexuality and children, the difficulties and potential for embarrassment and offence are redoubled.

Discussions of sexuality need to be clear about what aspects of sex are being examined. Firstly, of course, it is obvious that sex is a *biological fact* about human beings and their bodies. Humans have organs and body parts (genitals, breasts etc.) which are specialized and directly linked to the process of reproduction. There are other *secondary* sexual characteristics, such as body shape and body hair, which can be seen as arising out of our different reproductive roles and play a role in sexual attraction (Oakley 2005).

Secondly, we also use the word sex to describe a range of *activities* (sexual intercourse, oral sex, masturbation) which make use of these sexual characteristics, sometimes to bring about reproduction, sometimes solely for pleasure.

Thirdly, sex refers to a range of *social and personal meanings* given by people to the different things they do. We may ask whether an action is right or wrong. Is it sinful or holy? Is it consensual or forced? How does this action make me feel? Does it give me pleasure? What kinds of actions in what situations with what partners create desire in me?

This leads on to a fourth element of sexuality – that of *sexual orientation*. Are the objects of my sexual desire the same sex as me or different?

These four different aspects of sex and sexuality need to be separated because they have different implications for thinking about sex and its role in people's lives. For example, sex has an obvious function for the broader society. It seems clear that any society will need to find methods to control and schedule reproduction (Malinowski 1927). If a social group fails to reproduce, fails to create a new generation of people, it can die out. This may seem like a plot from a science fiction novel but, according to the anthropologist Colin Turnbull, such a fate did actually threaten the Ik, an East African tribe evicted from their ancestral lands who simply refused to reproduce in their new government-allocated homeland (Turnbull 1975). The 'social organization' of sex for reproduction is therefore a necessary feature of the ways in which societies operate.

Obviously, sex is not only something people engage in with the aim of reproducing the population. People engage in sexual activity for a huge variety of reasons and the 'real' reason may not be obvious to participants, let alone outsiders. With any sexual act, it is worth asking what the meaning of the act is to the different people involved. How do they think and feel about what is happening?

As Ken Plummer (1975) points out, the same set of actions (e.g. 'conventional' intercourse between a male and female adult) can have totally different significance depending on the different meanings the participants attribute to what is happening and their part in it. To an objective scientific observer the activity may be straightforward; certain parts of each body are moving and changing in certain ways which may be measurable and describable as a biological process. But Plummer points out that from the point of view of the two participants an enormous array of different things may be happening. We might ask any of the following questions: Are they both full, enthusiastic partners? Do they both feel that what is happening has the approval of their religion or personal morality? Has money (or some other favour) changed hands previously? Is one partner fantasizing about having sex with another person altogether? The answers to these questions might well transform our understanding of what is happening.

All societies have rules about what is acceptable and unacceptable in human sexual behaviour. These include rules about who are appropriate partners as well as what appropriate activities are (taboos on incest and laws about homosexuality, for example). Steven Box (1981), points out that in different states of the USA there have been laws against fornication, adultery, oral sex, masturbation, sodomy, and even sex with the light on! Societies frequently see ungoverned and unregulated sex as a threat to social order and frequently see that there is a need to repress sexual activity as a way of re-channelling energy towards other purposes, such as survival or fighting. The rules about sex vary from time to time and from culture to culture. It does seem to be the case that all known societies have had taboos on incest (Levi-Strauss 1947), but the precise application of this rule varies enormously from society to society – both the kinds of relatives who are forbidden partners and those who are allowed, or even in some cases where kinship rules insist you marry a person from a precise category, required. For example, in some cultures a man marrying his brother's widow would be incestuous while in others it would be what was required of him.

Activity 2.3.1: Childhood and sexuality

Consider the following points and write down your responses to them:

- Are children sexual beings?
- When does sexuality begin?
- Why is the association of sexuality and childhood such a taboo subject?

Sexuality and children

If we can generally identify sexuality as an area where social norms and reactions tend to be powerfully enforced this is even more the case for any situations which associate children and sexuality. Sexuality plays a vital role in popular thinking about childhood largely because in many societies it is absent from definitions of childhood's 'true' nature. Part of the ideal of childhood innocence is the idea of the asexual child. Associating children with sexuality runs up against some of the most forceful and significant social taboos.

Postman, whose account of the history of childhood is strongly influenced by the work of Ariès, argues that the idea of 'shame' is at the heart of changes in our conception of childhood and that this centres substantially on 'adults keeping secrets' from children. These secrets are largely sexual. In what Postman describes as the 'Dark Ages' and the Middle Ages, there was an openness about sexuality and sexual behaviour even in the presence of children. 'The idea of concealing sexual drives was alien to adults and the idea of sheltering children from sexual secrets unknown' (Postman 1994: 17). Orme points out that 'In homes where privacy was often restricted, young people must have become aware of the sexual activity of adults sooner than happens today ... Many adults, it seems were not concerned to keep their offspring innocent of such matters' (Orme 2001: 328).

Postman goes on to argue that the coming of literacy and the associated 'separation of mind and body' led writers to begin to stress the role of 'shame', of decorous behaviour and self-control and for adults the central importance of keeping secrets from the young: '... secrets about sexual relations, but also about money, about violence about illness, about death, about social relations. There even developed language secrets – that is a store of words not to be spoken in the presence of children' (Postman 1994: 49).

This process culminated in what may be seen as the nineteenth-century image of the innocent child who needed to be protected from adult knowledge and corruption. For the Victorians the idealized view of childhood excluded sex and sexuality. Children were generally seen as pure and asexual. In many ways this reflected the Victorian view of respectable women, who were seen as having no sexual desire and were encouraged to surrender to sex as a necessary submission to their husband's 'animal' desires ('lie back and think of England!'). Active sexuality was seen as the prerogative of adult males and fallen women (Marcus 1966). This idealization of childhood seemed to be completely compatible with a world where the recruitment of such 'fallen' women could take place at a very young age:

> A Royal Commission in 1871 found that in three London hospitals there were 2,700 cases of venereal disease among girls between the ages of 11 and 16 years. The sexual use of young girls was indirectly sanctioned as 12 was the age of consent. Girls of this age could be procured for the (substantial) price of £20, a valuation which gave some clue to the social class of the purchasers.
>
> (Hawkes 1996: 47)

Children's lack of any form of sexuality was a taken-for-granted aspect of their lives. Yet paradoxically, it was also something which needed to be enforced by social rules. The classic example of this attempt to force asexuality upon children, especially boys, was the Victorian moral campaign against masturbation. This was a long-term campaign that brought together some religious writers, whose beliefs led them to see any kind of physical pleasure not linked to procreation as something inherently sinful, with doctors and early psychologists who began to suggest that there were dire personal and social consequences resulting from the practice. Masturbation was seen as leading to imbecility, mental illness and infertility, as well as a general lack of moral strength (Weeks 1989). As Comfort (1968) points out, this led to a range of painful techniques to restrain children identified as in danger of engaging in 'self-abuse', including physical implements fitted to the body and brutal punishments for transgression (Porter and Hall 1995).

Freud and childhood sexuality

As this atmosphere of Victorian repression carried over into the beginning of the twentieth century it is not surprising that the ideas of Sigmund Freud (1986 [1905]) about childhood sexuality met with horror and incredulity. Writing in Vienna when it was still one of the twin capitals of the Hapsburg Empire, Freud put forward the view that sexuality was not something which came suddenly to children at some point shortly after puberty along with body hair and acne. Freud argued that children are born with the capacity for sexual pleasure, but that this is a capacity dispersed throughout the body – children can take sexual pleasure from all kinds of touch, stimulation, tickling etc. and from all parts of the body (mouth, anus, nipples, toes). Freud's model of 'normal' sexual development saw this generalized capacity for pleasure ('polymorphous perversity') gradually channelled into reproduction. So, for boys, the key site of sexual pleasure becomes the penis, while for girls it centres on the womb. Freud's theory was shocking and truly revolutionary in that it undermined the Victorian image of asexual childhood. More than that, it suggested that our adult sexuality was an artefact, a socio-biological creation generated by the ways in which we bring up children. Our sexual identity came to be seen as an outcome of the dynamics of family life, and some writers influenced by Freud perceived that this might result in other possible sexualities.

It is clear that modern audiences are much less shocked by Freud's ideas partly because during the twentieth century much of the thinking of Freudians and other writers about sexuality became gradually incorporated into 'common-sense' views about sexual life. Ideas about the key influence of early experience, the negative consequences of repression and the links between sexual behaviour and good mental and physical health became part of everyday language. They were powerful influences on theorists of childcare such as John Bowlby (1953) and writers of advisory books like Benjamin Spock (1979). Although Freud himself was politically and socially relatively conservative, his ideas had an influence on wider social and interpersonal changes across the twentieth century. Their broader impact was often seen a having played a role in bringing about the 'permissive' era of the 1960s, where there was a general tendency in advanced industrial societies like Britain, France and the US, to accept that people should be tolerant of other's preferences and orientations. As the hippy slogan said, 'Whatever turns you on!'

Activity 2.3.2: Freud and sexuality

- Read Freud (1986) [1905] *On Sexuality: Three Essays on the Theory of Sexuality and Other Works*, Harmondsworth: Penguin Books.
- Summarize Freud's description of childhood sexuality.
- What is your response to Freud's ideas – do you think they have any credibility?

The 1960s and reactions to them

Of course no society changes quite as suddenly and completely as might be suggested by Philip Larkin in his poem 'Annus Mirabilis', which begins 'Sexual intercourse began / In 1963 ... / Between the end of the Chatterley ban / And the Beatles' first LP' and it is important to stress that the 1960s were not always as permissive in sexual terms as some people suggest. Nevertheless this decade, when homosexuality and abortion were (partially) legalized and contraception became widely available, later came to be seen by many writers, particularly those associated with the New Right of the 1980s, as the source of the majority of those social problems that seemed to afflict Western society. In Britain many thought these problems could only be solved by a return to *traditional rules* or, in the words of Margaret Thatcher, 'Victorian values' (these Victorian values never seemed to include the nineteenth century's vast industry of prostitution and child sexual slavery, incidentally). Rolling back what was seen as the 1960s tide of sexual liberalism was at the forefront of this movement, and the sexual behaviour of the young was the key target. A first goal was to combat what was identified by some critics as a movement within education to 'promote' homosexuality among children.

Freudians and other psychoanalysts have tended to stress the extent to which sexuality is socially constructed rather than as something determined completely by the logic of biological necessity. Such a view sees the ways in which children are treated and the patterns of relationships they engage in as critical for how they develop a sexual identity. This gives particular significance to debates about choice of sexual orientation. If people realize that they are predominantly attracted to people of the same sex, then psychoanalytic theories would suggest that this arises from processes which take place very early in life. Therefore, it could be argued that much of the alarm about 'vulnerable' adolescents being seduced into homosexuality by predatory adults is misplaced. The problem with Section 28 – the clause in the 1988 Local Government Act which outlawed the 'promotion' of homosexuality in schools – can then be seen as the way in which it seemed to contribute to stopping teachers from responding appropriately to adolescents' emerging awareness of their own sexual preferences. It was not about protecting impressionable youth from being 'led astray'; rather it was concerned with the ability of teachers to respond to the needs of their pupils in an appropriate way (Durham 1991). Nevertheless the debate about the proper role of schooling in channelling or supporting children's ability to determine their own sexual preferences was dominated for a long period by the debate about Section 28 (Stonewall 2003).

In more recent years there has been a shift of focus brought about by the adoption in many schools of equal opportunities policies which single out homophobia along with racism, sexism etc. as unacceptable. This development of policy sits less well with the growing awareness of the problem of homophobic bullying (Douglas, *et al.* 1999; Hunt and Jensen 2007). Research in schools finds evidence of a high incidence of verbal and physical attacks on pupils identified as gay or lesbian and many barriers to schools being able to deal with the issues raised. It seems clear then that children who are trying to make sense of their sexual identity face a high level of potential hostility and in many cases a lack of support from the institutions they are in.

> ### Case study: Homophobic bullying in schools
>
> According to the pressure group Stonewall in their document *The School Report* (2007):
>
> - Almost two thirds (65 per cent) of young lesbian, gay and bisexual people experience homophobic bullying in school.
> - Almost three in five (58 per cent) of those experiencing bullying never report it but, if they do tell a teacher, 62 per cent of the time nothing is done.
> - Half of teachers fail to respond to homophobic language when they hear it.
> - Only a quarter of schools say that homophobic bullying is wrong in their school; in those schools gay young people are 60 per cent more likely not to have been bullied.
> - Homophobia and homophobic bullying are major problems for pupils, parents, staff and all those involved with young people and their education, irrespective of whether they are straight, lesbian, gay, bisexual or trans.
> - Homophobic bullying is not only experienced by pupils or professionals who are lesbian, gay or bisexual. It can also affect any child, young person or staff member who does not conform to ways of behaving that are traditionally associated with being 'masculine' or 'feminine'. Abuse can be verbal, physical or psychological.
>
> - Why is there a difference in approach to homophobia as compared with issues like racism and sexism?
> - What kinds of approach to problems of homophobic bullying can different educational institutions take?
>
> *The School Report* is available online at: http://www.stonewall.org.uk/documents/school_report.pdf

Conclusion: sexuality, sexual behaviour and social control

A consistent thread throughout the discussions above has been the link between people's ideas of sexuality and childhood and their models of social order and a controlled society. There is seen to be a clear connection between how we deal with children's sexuality and the broader issues of the kind of adult society we are aiming to construct.

According to Michel Foucault (1979), control of sexuality is closely related to the forms of social life created by modern rational technological society. He argued that the development of a society which is increasingly rationally administered needed to be based on control of people's bodies, and this was put into effect especially through the medicalization of aspects of our bodily life which had previously been seen as private. Medicalization took aspects of our bodies and our intimate lives and subjected them to outside scrutiny. At the heart of this process was a new approach to sex. Foucault rejects the view that Victorians were 'not interested' in sex. On the contrary, he argues they were centrally concerned with it as a focus for controlling people's lives. Foucault (1979: 26) says of the beginning of this attention in the seventeenth century, 'Sex became an issue, and a public issue no less; a whole web of discourses, special knowledges, analyses and injunctions settled upon it'.

This need to scrutinize and control people's bodies becomes a key element of developing forms of social control and focuses on children. We can see this in nineteenth-century campaigns on masturbation culminating in the element of the Boy Scout Oath of 1911 which states:

A SCOUT IS CLEAN IN THOUGHT, WORD AND DEED. Decent Scouts look down upon silly youths who talk dirt, and they do not let themselves give way to temptation, either to talk it or to do anything dirty. A Scout is pure, and clean-minded, and manly.

(Baden Powell 1911)

A similar approach is implied in later calls for the return of Victorian values, through to current concerns about the sexualization of media for pre-teens. Most recently the sexual content of magazines for young people has been described as too explicit by some, but as a genuine reflection of what young people know and need to know by others (Rush and La Nauze 2006).

Thus it is impossible to separate arguments about sexuality from broader debates about the rights of children and the role of adult power in controlling their lives. Controversies about homophobia, the age of consent, contraceptive advice to under 16s and sex education in schools all centre on competing images of childhood as vulnerable and dependent, characterized by an innocence requiring protection, as against a perspective which stresses children's rights as citizens able to decide for themselves and take greater responsibility for their own choices and their consequences (Corteen and Scraton 1997).

In the era of HIV/AIDS this is a major issue for those working with the young. It is important to place initiatives on sexual behaviour and sexual health within a context of the experience of childhood and adolescence as they are currently experienced. As Moore and Rosenthal (1993: 4) put it, 'Education about sexual values and sexual health is likely to be most effective if educators take into account the current beliefs and practices of their target audience'. Thus the need to accord children a right to be heard and a recognition of their own preferences and orientations are likely to underpin the most effective strategies to protect their health and well-being.

Student reflection

One of the aims of this chapter is to inform you about issues to do with sexuality. As far as children are concerned, they have the right to appropriate sex education.

* Consider the way that you think children should be informed about sex in school. Do you think you had appropriate and useful sex education at school?

Key points

* Sex and sexuality can be extremely emotive topics of discussion, particularly in relation to childhood.
* Sexuality has many aspects: biological (reproduction and attraction), activities (e.g. sexual intercourse/masturbation for pleasure as well as reproduction), social/personal meanings (e.g. sinful, consensual) and sexual orientation.
* It can be argued that sex is part of 'social organization' (i.e. societies need to control reproduction) and has social rules which can vary according to cultural values.
* Contemporary thinking is that sexuality is not synonymous with childhood, instead childhood is represented as innocent (the asexual child). However, historically this was not the case.
* Postman (1994) suggests that historically the growth of literacy led writers to discuss

and promote 'shame' and the need for adults to keep secrets about sex (plus money, death, illness etc.).
- Victorian England saw childhood sexuality enforced by social rules such as the campaign against masturbation which suggested that it was sinful and harmful.
- Freud suggested that instead of children being asexual, children are born with the capacity for sexual pleasure.
- More recent debates have surrounded sexual orientation including 'Section 28' which outlawed the 'promotion' of homosexuality in schools. Research in schools finds evidence of much homophobic bullying in schools.
- It could be questioned as to how young people's sexual health and behaviour can be improved without listening and responding to their own identified needs.

Recommended reading

Corteen, K. and Scraton, P. (1997) Prolonging childhood, manufacturing 'innocence' and regulating sexuality, in P. Scraton (ed.) *Childhood in Crisis*, London: UCL Press.
Gittins, D. (1998) *The Child in Question*, London: Macmillan.
Nye, R. A. (1999) *Sexuality*, Oxford: Oxford University Press.

References

Baden Powell (1911). 'A scout is clean in thought, word and deed.' Quoted in: The Inquiry Net (2003) Scout Law History. Available online at: http://www.inquiry.net/ideals/scout_law/chart.htm (accessed 7.9.2009).
Bowlby, J. (1953) *Child Care and the Growth of Love*, Harmondsworth: Penguin Books.
Box, S. (1981) *Deviance, Reality and Society*, London: Halt Rinehart Winston.
Comfort, A. (1968) *The Anxiety Makers*, London: Pantheon.
Corteen, K. and Scraton, P. (1997) Prolonging childhood, manufacturing 'innocence' and regulating sexuality, in P. Scraton (ed.) *Childhood in Crisis*, London: UCL Press.
Douglas, N., Warwick, I., Whitty, G., Aggleton, P. and Kemp, S. (1999) Homophobic bullying in secondary schools in England and Wales – teachers' experiences, *Health Education*, 99 (2): 53–60.
Durham, M. (1991) *Sex and Politics: The Family and Morality in the Thatcher Years*, London: Macmillan.
Foucault, M. (1979) *The History of Sexuality: Vol. 1: An Introduction*, Harmondsworth: Penguin Books.
Freud, S. (1986) [1905] *On Sexuality: Three Essays on the Theory of Sexuality and Other Works*, Harmondsworth: Penguin Books.
Hawkes, G. (1996) *A Sociology of Sex and Sexuality*, Buckingham: Open University Press.
Hunt, R. and Jensen, J. (2007) *The School Report: The Experiences of Young Gay People in Britain's Schools*, London: Stonewall. Available online at: http://www.stonewall.org.uk/documents/school_report.pdf
Levi-Strauss, C. (1977) [1947] *Elementary Structures of Kinship*, new edn, London: Beacon Press.
Malinowski, B. (1927) *Sex and Repression in Savage Society*, London: Routledge.
Marcus, S. (1966) *The Other Victorians: A Study of Sexuality and Pornography in Mid-Nineteenth Century England*, London: Book Club Associates.
Moore, S. and Rosenthal, D. (1993) *Sexuality in Adolescence*, London: Routledge.
Oakley, A. (2005) *The Ann Oakley Reader: Gender Women and Social Science*, London: Policy Press.
Orme, N. (2001) *Medieval Children*, New Haven: Yale University Press
Plummer, K. (1975) *Sexual Stigma: An Interactionist Account*, London: Routledge.

Porter, R. and Hall, L. (1995) *The Facts of Life: The Creation of Sexual Knowledge in Britain 1650–1950*, New Haven: Yale University Press.

Postman, N. (1994) *The Disappearance of Childhood*, New York: Vintage.

Rush, E and La Nauze, A. (2006) *Corporate Paedophilia – Sexualisation of Children in Australia*, The Australia Institute Discussion Paper No. 90. Available online at: https://www.tai.org.au/file.php?file=DP90.pdf

Spock, B. (1979) *Baby and Child-Care*, 4th edn, Oxford: Bodley.

Stonewall (2003) The School Report. Available online at: http://www.stonewall.org.uk/documents/school_report.pdf (accessed 7.9.2009).

Turnbull, C. (1975) *The Mountain People*, London: Picador.

Weeks, J. (1989) *Sex, Politics and Society: The Regulation of Sexuality since 1800*, 2nd edn, London: Longman.

Part 3

Children and risk

Part 3 of this publication deals with areas of childhood and life experiences of children and young people which can put them 'at risk' – risk being defined in Kennedy's chapter, citing Jaeger, *et al.* (2001: 17), as any situation, event or occasion in which something of human value – including themselves – is at stake.

Kennedy highlights the fact that in contemporary society, due to modern definitions of harm and how to avoid it, we are beset with moral panics concerning a plethora of potential risks from CJD ('mad cow disease') to child abuse. In keeping with Robinson (Chapter 4.1, this volume), Kennedy comments on the role of the media in creating and spreading these moral panics.

Kennedy goes on to consider how fear of risk can be potentially harmful to society in general as the public's cry for protection from risks, encouraging governmental intervention, can produce the nanny state scenario. In terms of the development of children, too much caution can be detrimental and can limit their opportunities for new experiences, even to the extent of not being allowed to play outdoors. Kennedy concludes that while risk can not be eliminated, it should be carefully managed so as not to interfere with the confidence, self-esteem and physical, mental and emotional well-being of children (Edgington 2007).

Clearly, one of the most significant areas where children may be 'at risk' is that of abuse – be it physical, emotional or sexual. While highlighting the difficulties in defining and detecting child abuse, Kendall, with reference to some recent, high-profile cases, categorizes the many different forms that abuse can take. She comments on the difficulties of detecting child abuse due to the fact that the majority of perpetrators of abuse are adults known and trusted by the children involved. Moreover, she points out that policies and initiatives put in place by governments to safeguard children, such as the CRB check and the *Every Child Matters* agenda in the UK, are not failsafe. While suggesting that child abuse can never be completely eliminated, Kendall concludes that in order to limit instances of abuse, much more effective inter-agency and inter-disciplinary working and information sharing is required.

Kassem's chapter exploring the social world of looked-after children suggests that for far too long those social systems which have placed children 'at risk' within their home environments have focused on individual stereotypes such a 'the bad parent' or 'the troublesome kid'. Kassem asserts that if we are serious about improving the life chances of looked-after children we must examine larger socio-economic structures. In line with Grant's chapter (Chapter 4.4, this volume), Kassem believes that poverty is one of the key factors which affects looked-after children throughout their lifespans. In a sense, many children end up being looked after, whether that be in residential care or in foster homes, due to poverty within in the familial home and the continuum of consequences of poverty ranging from an inability to provide for children to stress and mental health issues and, at worst, to neglect, abuse, criminal activity and addiction. Once children are within the care system they often experience poverty in terms of lack of ownership, not just of material possessions, but also of a sense of well-being and belonging. This cycle of poverty, coupled by low educational achievement, continues for many looked-after children once they leave the care system and enter the adult world. Kassem suggests that if we really want to tackle the issues faced by looked-after children, we must break the cycle of child poverty and we must improve the structure and organization of the care system. Too often residential and foster care breaks down due to poor financing and resourcing and an inexperienced and poorly qualified workforce.

Harrison's chapter highlights the important difference between mental health, which we all have, hopefully in terms of mental well-being, and mental illness which is a complex topic encompassing a number of causes and disorders. Harrison outlines the potential causes of mental illness in the young, such as birth factors, physical disease or injury and environmental factors, and the disorders, whether developmental, emotional, affective, attentional or conduct-based, which can result from mental ill health. Harrison also notes the social stigmas which are associated with mental illness and, in line with Foucault (2006), he points out the fact that mental health is frequently defined in socio-historical and cultural terms. To conclude, Harrison considers how mental ill health in the young is treated in the UK today, pointing out some of the issues related to this treatment such as the level of specialism, or lack thereof, of professionals, the length of time children must wait for treatment and the frequency with which treatment is not taken up or followed through.

References

Edgington, M. (2007) Supporting young children to engage with risk and challenge, *Early Years Update*, May.

Foucault, M. (2006) [1961] *The History of Madness*, London: Routledge.

Jaeger, C. C., Renn, O., Rosa, E. A., and Webler, T. (2001) *Risk, Uncertainty, and Rational Action*, London: Earthscan Publications.

3.1   Children and the notion of risk

The nanny state?

Andrew Kennedy

Between 1970–2 and 2000–2, the death rate (all causes) for boys in England and Wales aged 0–4 years fell from 4.6 per thousand to 1.4 per thousand; for boys aged 5–9 years it fell from 0.4 per thousand to 0.1 per thousand. The number of girls dying fell by roughly the same proportion over the same period (ONS 2007). The rate of *accidental* deaths among all children aged 0–14 in England and Wales fell from 18 per 100,000 in 1971 to 5 per 100,000 in 1995 (ONS 1997). It is clear that children's lives are becoming safer by the year.

This is very far from the picture which is portrayed by the press and broadcasters. More than ever before, government policy is directed at protecting children who are considered to be 'at risk'; the *Every Child Matters* Green Paper explicitly replaced the policy of focusing attention on those children who were deemed to be most vulnerable with a system in which all children were to be kept under close surveillance lest they come to harm (DfES 2003).

Activity 3.1.1: Defining risk

Consider the following questions and write down your responses.

- How would you define 'risk'?
- What are the risks that children in contemporary society face?
- Are these risks any different from those faced by children in previous times?
- Can risk be a good thing?

Jaeger, *et al.* (2001: 17) define risk as follows: 'a situation or event in which something of human value (including humans themselves) has been put at stake and where the outcome is uncertain.' They make the point that risk offers both dangers and opportunities; there are 'good' and 'bad' risks, as well as those which are simply taken for granted or ignored. For example, in the United Kingdom in 2002 there were 96,489 reported accidents involving children (RoSPA 2004). Of these, by far the greatest number (43,011) took place in the home, and yet parents increasingly choose to keep their children indoors for fear of what might happen to them outside. In 2004, the *Observer* reported:

> [A] survey of more than 1,000 children aged 10 and 11 reveals that the choice to remain indoors is being made because of an increasingly unrealistic assessment by children and their parents of the risks of the outside world .... The survey found that

danger was the first thing children mentioned when talking about being outside, citing a fear of strangers as reason for not playing outside, believing they faced a high risk of being kidnapped, murdered, or sexually assaulted.

(*Observer* 2004)

In fact, the number of children being killed by another person (homicide) has remained largely unchanged since the 1970s: in 2005–6, 55 children were homicide victims in England and Wales. In 44 per cent of these cases, the principal suspects were the victims' own parents, and another 24 per cent were family members, friends, or acquaintances. Only 22 per cent of victims were known to have been killed by strangers, while 11 per cent of the killers were unidentified. Of the cases in which parents were suspected, there was a near-balance between mothers (47 per cent) and fathers (53 per cent) (NSPCC 2007a). Furthermore, in 2002–3, 68 children in England and Wales were known to have been successfully abducted by strangers, which represents just 9 per cent of all recorded child abductions (NSPCC 2007b).

The statistics would appear to show, then, that children have more to fear from their own families than from strangers, and that the home is a more dangerous place to be than almost anywhere else. How has it come to be that parents' fears about the risks that face their children are so misplaced?

Banishing risk

Lupton (1999) shows how the modernist conception of risk arose from a desire to use reason to banish the earlier view of the world as an uncertain, unpredictable place. Instead, the world becomes manageable through what Reddy (1996, cited in Lupton 1999: 7) describes as 'the myth of calculability' – in other words, if we can only take all factors into account we can establish exactly what level of risk we face in a particular situation and then take measures to nullify it. This view makes the very large (and unproven) assumption that all factors can be identified and quantified. However, by the end of the twentieth century, the idea of there being both good and bad risks had become replaced by the word's association with danger; for most people, risk thus becomes a negative concept.

Illich takes this view a step further:

> Progress in civilization became synonymous with the reduction in the sum total of suffering. From then on, politics was taken to be an activity not so much for maximising happiness as for minimising pain. The result is a tendency to see pain as essentially a passive happening inflicted on helpless victims because the toolbox [i.e. the means available to government] ... is not being used in their favour .... In this context ... it seems reasonable to eliminate pain, even at the cost of losing independence.

(Illich 1976: 151–2)

In referring to pain, Illich is including broader ideas of illness, affliction, distress, and even sadness, hunger and tiredness. His concern is that as society intervenes increasingly to mitigate pain, whether by medical intervention or by other means, so the individual loses the ability to cope with reality and instead begins to interpret every ache as an indicator of their 'need for padding or pampering' (Illich 1976: 133). Whereas Western society previously attempted to achieve more accuracy in predicting the outcome of events, it now concerns itself increasingly with avoiding all unpleasant sensations or outcomes.

The suggestion that people are increasingly treated as helpless victims is developed by Furedi (2002: 170–1), who identifies a number of factors in this process. He cites the influence of biology, for example the influence of hormones leading to undesirable male behaviour. He also examines the power of the belief in the social causation of many problems – the idea that people are made to act as they do because of factors such as poverty, particular cultural or class values, and poor education. The result of these and other factors is a growing tendency to assume that individuals are powerless to control their own fates, a sense of powerlessness which is accentuated by societal changes which have led to a loss of social solidarity (one could note the increasing reluctance of adults either to correct misbehaviour by children they encounter in public places, or even to assist children who are obviously in distress). In these circumstances people become vulnerable to claims of every alleged new danger, and their belief in their own powerlessness leads them to demand that someone in 'authority' do something to protect them.

People who are professionally involved in caring for children are very aware of changing public attitudes towards risk. The loss of trust between welfare professionals and the public, along with the government's emphasis on targets and accountability, has led to social workers in particular taking a pessimistic view of any potential risks to children (Wyness 2006). There is also fear of what has been described as the 'compensation culture'. A House of Commons Committee found that '... there is plenty of evidence of excessive risk aversion and a mistaken perception that it is caused by litigation' (House of Commons 2006: 13). The report cited Gaskin (2005) as saying that public caution was being fuelled by media reports (House of Commons 2006: 15), and it drew particular attention to the way such caution was restricting children's freedom. It specifically identified the target-setting culture in public life as a source of excessive caution: by setting numerical targets for the reduction in the number of accidents, rather than ensuring that reasonable measures are taken to reduce risk, the tendency is to stop completely any potentially risky activities.

> The Health and Safety Executive admitted that it was unable to conduct risk balancing exercises looking at the dangers of different risks ... [but the Committee stressed that] responsible risk management does not equate to the avoidance of all risk.
>
> (House of Commons 2006: 18)

Moral panics

Mike Campbell, Professor of Medical Statistics at Sheffield University, explains that the general public tend to have a very poor understanding of risk, and he makes the point that risks are subject to fashion, citing meningitis, necrotizing fasciitis (the 'flesh-eating bug'), CJD ('mad cow disease') and listeria as examples of diseases which caught the imagination of press and public, and of which, for a time, every case was reported (notice the dramatic labels which the media attach to some of these conditions). The other example he gives is the fear of child molesters and the effect which it has had on children's school and social activities, despite the lack of evidence that children are at any greater risk than they were 50 years ago (Campbell 1999). Fashions such as these can develop into full-blown moral panics.

Moral panics are campaigns which 'appeal to people who are alarmed by an apparent fragmentation or breakdown of the social order, which leaves them at risk in some way .... Politicians and some parts of the media are eager to lead [these campaigns] to have action taken that they claim would suppress the threat' (Thompson 1998: 3–5). An example of this would be what Jenkins (1998: 127) describes as 'the rediscovery of the issue of sexual offences against children' in the United States of America. He shows how increased sensitivity to the issue led to changes in the law on reporting sexual abuse, which in turn resulted in a surge of up to 3,000 per cent in the number of cases being reported. By 1990 there were claims in the press that child abuse had risen by 80 per cent in ten years, and child sexual abuse had risen by 277 per cent, whereas what had actually increased was people's willingness to come forward and talk about such incidents. This gave rise to a belief that there was an epidemic of abuse. As interest in the issue increased, the definition of sexual abuse was broadened, which in turn further increased the number of cases being reported. This is by no means the same as saying that more children were suffering than had been the case a decade previously.

Hidden agendas

'Then what can you want to do now?' said the old lady, gaining courage. 'I wants to make your flesh creep,' replied the boy.

(Charles Dickens, *The Pickwick Papers*)

There is a range of interest groups which stand to gain from a growing climate of fear. For example, there is money to be made: Madeleine McCann disappeared from a holiday apartment in Portugal on 3 May 2007, and from then until the end of July 2008 there were 919 articles about her published in the *Daily Mail* alone – more than two every day (*Daily Mail* 2008). It was a story with many intriguing aspects, but however sad the events were they did only concern one child, yet the constant repetition and embellishment of the details served to keep it in the public mind for more than a year. It also sold a lot of newspapers.

Groups campaigning for particular causes (sometimes called single-issue groups) are competing with each other for publicity, money and, often, legislative time. They need to make their arguments stand out, and one good way to do this is to produce some dramatic (and often alarming) statistics. This can produce a disproportionate impression of the scale of the problem. 'When advocacy groups use surveys to draw attention to their causes the reported change – however extreme the organization may make it sound – is often from small to slightly less small' (Glassner 1999: 119). The 'epidemic' of child sexual abuse could be seen as an example of this phenomenon, if indeed there was any increase at all. In fact, the proportion of calls to Childline (UK) which related to sexual abuse fell from 27 per cent in 1986–7 (ONS 1997: 151) to 7 per cent in 2002–3 (ONS 2004: 129). The greatest increases concerned relationship problems and bullying.

Sometimes the facts are simply too uncomfortable to express in a culture which prides itself on being 'non-judgemental':

Children of parents who have never worked or who are long-term unemployed are 13 times more likely to die from unintentional injury, and 37 times more likely to die as a result of exposure to smoke, fire, and flames than children of parents in higher managerial and professional occupations.

(DCSF 2008: 60)

It could be questioned as to how much more comforting it is to be able to look outwards and blame negligent social workers, or unsafe playgrounds and roads, or anonymous strangers, than for individual families to confront their problems.

Governments can sometimes legislate in response to a public outcry which follows a sensational news story. An example of this is the Soham murders of 2002, in which two schoolgirls were murdered by a school caretaker. A direct result of this was a judicial inquiry (the Bichard Inquiry) which led to the passing of the Protection of Vulnerable Groups Act, 2006. This Act requires that all persons, professional or volunteer, who are involved in activities which bring them into contact with any people, young or old, who are deemed to be 'vulnerable', must undergo a Criminal Records Bureau check (Every Child Matters 2008a). O'Neill (2006) states that 'They used to say that it took a village to raise a child – today only state-sanctioned individuals will be allowed to raise a child. It takes a peculiarly paranoid state to infect children's minds with suspicion and adult minds with self-doubt'.

There is, too, a more calculated benefit to be gained by government from a climate of fear, and the demand that something should be done (almost regardless of what that something might be). The gathering and sharing of information about every member of the British population has been an important aspect of government policy since 1997, but there has been considerable public unease about this project, with concerns voiced both about the security of the personal data which is held and the uses to which it is being put. One outcome of the Children Act 2004 was the establishment of ContactPoint, a database which contains personal information about every child in England (Every Child Matters 2008b). ContactPoint was originally known as the Children's Information Sharing Database, but was re-branded because of public concerns about the sharing of so much personal information (ARCH 2008). In response to these concerns, the government delayed implementation of ContactPoint while a security review was conducted by the consultants Deloitte. The report's findings satisfied the Department for Children, Schools and Families that the project could go ahead, even though Deloitte had concluded that 'risk can only be managed not eliminated, and therefore there will always be a risk of data security incidents occurring' (*The Register* 2008a).

Every Child Matters made explicit the government's desire to remove legislative barriers which hindered the sharing of data between departments (DfES 2003: 10–11), and public resistance to such changes can be countered by stressing the dangers which children face and which will supposedly be lessened by taking such measures. ContactPoint is far from being the only children's database. ARCH points out that there are around 20 such databases, and that 'there are big questions over security and function creep, and of course at rock bottom it is a question of whether we can trust this government with any of our personal data' (*The Register* 2008b).

Consequences for children

> Always keep a-hold of Nurse
> For fear of finding something worse.
>> (Hilaire Belloc, 'Jim', from *Cautionary Tales*)

A recurring theme for several decades has been that of 'stranger danger', a message that is reinforced by respected sources such as schools (for example, Little Ridge CP School 2002), police forces (Gloucestershire 2008; Essex 2008; and others), and the BBC (2008a). As we have seen, the facts tell a very different story, but the unspecified, and thus all-encompassing notion of 'children at risk' implies that they are in constant danger, and this attitude becomes what Furedi (2001: 9–10) calls a 'cultural dogma' – an unchallenged truism. As Judith Gillespie, of the Scottish Parent Teacher Council, said, 'there is a danger we will de-skill children, and leave them unable to look out for their own safety and incapable of judging between risky and safe adults' (cited by O'Neill 2006).

This overcautious attitude to risk extends, however, far beyond emotive issues such as abduction and sexual molestation. In all activities where children are involved, adults are strongly encouraged to adopt the 'precautionary principle' – avoiding any activities or circumstances where the unexpected might happen, however unlikely it might seem. 'Intimidating public campaigns endlessly remind [parents] of the many risks their children face. It is difficult to retain a sense of perspective when the safety of children has become a permanent item of news' (Furedi 2001: 9–10).

Research conducted by Play England shows that only 29 per cent of children are allowed to play in natural outdoor environments, compared with 70 per cent of their parents' generation; 51 per cent of 7–12 year olds have been forbidden to climb trees without adult supervision. As the organization's Director, Adrian Voce, has said:

> Starting from their earliest play experiences, children both need and want to push their boundaries in order to explore their limits and develop their abilities. Children would never learn to walk, climb stairs or ride a bicycle unless they were strongly motivated to respond to challenges – but we must accept that these things inevitably involve an element of risk.
>
> Adventurous play that both challenges and excites children helps instil critical life skills. Constantly wrapping children in cotton wool can leave them ill equipped to deal with stressful or challenging situations they might encounter later in life.
>
> (Play England 2008)

There are consequences, too, for the behaviour and composition of the workforce: in many settings, carers are now forbidden from giving comforting hugs, while the workforce is becoming increasingly refeminized as men are driven out and the work is left to low-paid women (Glassner 1999: xvi). There has also been a marked reduction in the number of people coming forward to volunteer to work with children, whether in youth groups, sports clubs, or other activities, and one important reason for this is fear of litigation (House of Commons 2006: 16). Thus, children are denied what other societies would regard as normal contact with adults, and in particular are increasingly denied responsible male role models, and all this at a time when genuinely large numbers of children are suffering from deprivation, poor education, and poor home circumstances (Glassner 1999: xvii).

Finally, an overcautious approach to risk management can divert attention away from serious risks (House of Commons 2006: 14–15). This is one objection to using ContactPoint for identifying children who might be at risk of harm – rather than concentrating on a known number of individuals whose circumstances indicate specific threats, the responsible authorities are meant to be overseeing every child in the country, including the great majority who face no danger at all.

Activity 3.1.2: 'Good' and 'bad' risks

Choose an age group with which you might be working. Plan an activity which will take place in a semi-wild environment (think of woodland, grass, and a river or lake). The aim of the activity is to introduce the participants in an enjoyable way to experience risks which they might not previously have encountered.

You must undertake a detailed risk assessment, showing the risks (planned and unplanned) which you might encounter, the measures which you will take to minimize the danger to participants, and the benefits which they will gain from taking part. In order to do this successfully, you must distinguish clearly between 'good' and 'bad' risks and, as Furedi might put it, show what the participants can learn from the experience.

Discuss your plan with colleagues and see how far they agree with your assessment.

'Good' risks: the benefits of risk-taking

The Children's Play Council (2004) speaks of the importance of managing 'the balance between the need to offer risk and the need to keep children safe from harm'; it also stresses that unstructured and, at times, unsupervised play should be available. The Royal Society for the Prevention of Accidents has actually called for a 'massive increase' in opportunities for children to experience risk in order to prepare them for situations they will face later in life (RoSPA 2007).

The Department for Children, Schools and Families has come to recognize the harm to children's development which comes from spending excessive amounts of time in the home (DCSF 2008: 14), although its plans concentrate on providing managed outdoor play areas rather than giving freer access to the natural environment. It does, however, accept the need for children to learn to recognize and manage risk (DCSF 2008: 16).

The case for exposing children to greater challenges and to 'good' risk is put very clearly by Edgington (2007), who recognizes that the ability to assess and manage risk is important not just for a child's physical safety, but also for their confidence and self-esteem, and so for their mental and emotional well-being. She quotes Lindon (1999): 'Adults who assess every situation in terms of what could go wrong, risk creating anxiety in some children and recklessness in others.' Dwelling excessively on safety can, paradoxically, expose children to greater danger: 'Without challenges and risks, children will find play areas uninteresting or use them in inappropriate ways, which become dangerous' (Bilton 2005, cited by Edgington 2007). This is not to advocate a laissez-faire approach; Edgington stresses the need to distinguish between acceptable and unacceptable risks, to identify any children who need specific forms of support, and to establish clear expectations about behaviour. Parents must be involved in discussions about the process, too. The approach is summarized by Furedi (2001: 9–10) who suggests that rather than asking 'What can go wrong?' we should be asking 'Does it matter?' and 'What can the child learn from the experience?'

Case study: John Pinnington

Bingham (2008: 11) reports the following story:

A former vice-principal whose career was destroyed by unproven allegations of sex abuse has lost his attempt to have them wiped from his record.

John Pinnington, a father of two, was sacked from his job at a college for autistic adults when the claims, which he describes as 'fanciful and speculative', were disclosed in an enhanced criminal records check.

In a High Court case that could have consequences for thousands of carers working with children and vulnerable adults, he challenged a police decision to include the allegations on his extended criminal record certificate. But yesterday two judges concluded that the decision ... had not been 'unreasonable' despite 'strong doubt' over the veracity of the allegations.

[They] ruled that Mr. Pinnington's prospective employers 'should be aware' of the accusations, however weak and unreliable they were.

[A judge] added that despite how 'painful and damaging' disclosure might be, the law said that such information should be revealed to employers 'even if it only might be true'.

Mr. Pinnington ... was dismissed from his post in 2005 when a charity took over the college and ordered enhanced Criminal Records Bureau (CRB) checks.

[...]

His QC ... told the court that the allegations made by one of his accusers – a young man with autism who, she said, 'could not stop telling lies' because of his condition – were 'fanciful and speculative' and had been made to 'get attention'. ... But Lord Justice Richards concluded: '... nothing that happened after the police became involved was sufficient to establish that the original allegations could not be true ....'

Outside the court, Mr. Pinnington said the CRB certificate was 'based on lies' but had cost him 'my life and livelihood'. He said he had been jobless for three years as a result of the disclosures .... 'I want my life back,' he said.

In July, 2008, the BBC reported that 680 people had been wrongly labelled as criminals by the Criminal Records Bureau. The Home Office said that this was 'regrettable' and that this represented only 0.02 per of cases which the bureau had handled (BBC 2008b).

Having read the case study, and seen the effect that a disputed CRB check can have on a person's life, do you think that 680 is an acceptable number of people to have had their lives affected in this way?

Given the level of risk to children from their care workers as discussed in this chapter, how many errors of this kind do you think are a price worth paying in the attempt to ensure children's safety – more or fewer than 680?

Student reflection

Having read this chapter, return to the notes you made in response to Activity 3.1.1.

- Reconsider your responses to the question in Activity 3.1.1 – have your answers changed in any way?

Key points

- Not all risks are 'bad', the negative connotations of risk are due to a modern interpretation as avoiding 'harm'.
- Too much caution can be harmful to children and childhood and many children lack opportunities to play outdoors.
- It could be suggested that the interference of society to reduce risk leads to individuals who rely on the government and others for protection. This could mean that we become infantilized and lose our self-reliance.
- Moral panic can result from over-reporting and a climate of fear is profitable for the press.
- Risk aversion can be linked to fear of litigation.
- The government has tried to limit risk through workforce legislation such as CRB checks and ContactPoint but the reliability of this can be questioned.
- Risk can be managed but not eliminated.
- It is argued that children need to take risks and play unsupervised to grow, learn and to develop life skills such as overcoming challenges and developing confidence.

Recommended reading

Foucault, M. (1991) *Discipline and Punish: The Birth of the Prison*, new edn, Basingstoke: Penguin.
Furedi, F. (2002) *The Culture of Fear: Risk-taking and the Morality of Low Expectation*, New York and London: Continuum.
House of Commons, Constitutional Affairs Committee (2006) *Compensation Culture*, London: The Stationery Office.
Thompson, K. (1998) *Moral Panics*, London: Routledge.

References

ARCH (Action on Rights for Children) (2008) *'ContactPoint' – Formerly the Information Sharing Index*. Available online at: http://www.arch-ed.org/issues/databases/contactpoint.htm (accessed 7.8.2008).
BBC (2008a) 'Parenting: your kids – keeping them safe: stranger danger'. Available online at: http://www.bbc.co.uk/parenting/your_kids/safety_stranger.shtml (accessed 8.8.2008).
—— (2008b) 'Crime check errors "regrettable"'. Available online at http://news.bbc.co.uk/1/hi/uk/7491125.stm (accessed 5.7.2008).
Bingham J. (2008) 'Teacher's career is wrecked by "lies"'. *Daily Telegraph*, 1 August, p. 11.
Campbell, M. (1999) *Risk Communication*. Available online at: http://www.healthprotection.org.uk/ncbugs/Risk%20Communication.htm (accessed 7.8.2007).
Children's Play Council (2004) *Policy Position: The Importance of Good Play Provision*. Available online at: http://www.ncb.org.uk/dotpdf/open%20access%20-%20phase%201%only/policy objective_cpc_2004.pdf (accessed 31.7.2007).
Cohen, S. (1972) *Folk Devils and Moral Panics: The Creation of the Mods and Rockers*, London: MacGibbon & Kee.
Daily Mail (2008) Results for Madeleine McCann. Available online at: http://www.dailymail.co.uk/home/search.html?searchPhrase=madeleine+mccann (accessed 31.7.2008).
DCSF (Department for Children, Schools and Families) (2008) *Staying Safe: Action Plan*, Nottingham: DCSF Publications.
DfES (2003) *Every Child Matters: Summary*, Norwich: The Stationery Office.

Edgington, M. (2007) 'Supporting young children to engage with risk and challenge', *Early Years Update*, May.

Essex Police (2008) *Young People: Stranger Danger*. Available online at: http://www.essex.police.uk/offbeat/o_ki_02.php (accessed 8.8.2008).

Every Child Matters (2008a) *Independent Safeguarding Authority*. Available online at: http://www.everychildmatters.gov.uk/independentsafeguardingauthority/ (accessed 7.8.2008).

—— (2008b) *ContactPoint*. Available online at: http://www.everychildmatters.gov.uk/delivering-services/contactpoint/ (accessed 7.8.2008).

—— (2008c) *Every Child Matters: Change for Children – Home*. Available online at: http://www.everychildmatters.gov.uk/ (accessed 27.7.2007).

Foucault, M. (1991) *Discipline and Punish: The Birth of the Prison*, new edn, Basingstoke: Penguin.

Furedi, F. (2001) *Paranoid Parenting: Abandon Your Anxieties and be a Good Parent*, London: Penguin.

—— (2002) *The Culture of Fear: Risk-taking and the Morality of Low Expectation*, New York and London: Continuum.

Glassner, B. (1999) *The Culture of Fear: Why Americans are Afraid of the Wrong Things*, New York: Basic Books.

Gloucestershire Police (2008) *Kids Aware: Stranger Danger*. Available online at: http://www.gloucestershire.police.uk/kids_aware/3.html (accessed 8.8.2008).

House of Commons, Constitutional Affairs Committee (2006) *Compensation Culture*, London: The Stationery Office.

Illich, I. (1976) *Limits to Medicine: Medical Nemesis: The Expropriation of Health*, London: Marion Boyars.

Jaeger, C. C., Renn, O., Rosa, E. A. and Webler, T. (2001) *Risk, Uncertainty, and Rational Action*, London: Earthscan Publications.

Jenkins, P. (1998) *Moral Panic: Changing Concepts of the Child Molester in Modern America*, New Haven, CT and London: Yale University Press.

Lindon, J. (2007) 'Are children too safe for their own good?', *Practical Pre-School*, April: pp. 6–7.

Little Ridge CP School (2002) *Be Safe – Say NO! to Strangers*. Available online at: http://ww.littleridge.e-sussex.sch.uk/2002/Summer2002/StrangerDanger/besfe.htm (accessed 31.7.2006).

Lupton, D. (1999) *Risk*, London: Routledge.

NSPCC (2007a) *Child Homicides: Key Protection Statistics (December 2007)*. Available online at: http://www.nspcc.org.uk/Inform/resourcesforprofessionals/Statistics/KeyCPStats/4_wda48747.html (accessed 31.7.2008).

—— (2007b) *Child Abductions: Key Protection Statistics (December 2007)*. Available online at: http://www.nspcc.org.uk/Inform/resourcesforprofessionals/Statistics/KeyCPStats/15_wda48733.html (accessed 31.7.2008).

O'Neill, B. (2006) 'Heavy vetting', *Guardian*, 25.10.2006.

Observer (2004) '"Stranger danger" drive harms kids'. Available online at: http://www.guardian.co.uk/politics/2004/may/23/uk.children (accessed 31.7.2008).

ONS (Office for National Statistics) (1997) *Social Trends 27*, London: The Stationery Office.

—— (2004) *Social Trends 34*, London: The Stationery Office.

—— (2007) *Annual Abstracts of Statistics 143*, Basingstoke: Palgrave Macmillan.

Play England (2008) *New Figures for Playday 2008 Reveal Children Deprived of Adventurous Play*. Available online at: http://www.playengland.org.uk/Page.asp?originx_7663lg_88857648193x4s_200883188v (accessed 4.8.2008).

Rich, D. (2007) 'Real-life risk', *Nursery Education*, January, pp. 14–15.

RoSPA (2004) *Child Accident Statistics*. Available online at: http://www.rospa.com/factsheets/child_accidents.pdf (accessed 31.7.2008).

—— (2007) *RoSPA Press Release: More Schemes Needed to Help Children Experience Risk*, Birmingham: Royal Society for the Prevention of Accidents.

The Register (2008a) 'Deloitte flags risks of UK child database'. Available online at: http://www.theregister.co.uk/2008/02/22/child_database_review/ (accessed 7.8.2008).

—— (2008b) 'Government wants every English child on "secure" database'. Available online at: http://www.theregister.co.uk/2008/02/13/england_child_database/ (accessed 7.8.2008).

Thompson, K. (1998) *Moral Panics*, London: Routledge.

Woonton, M. (2006) 'Taking risks is vital for providing truly inclusive practice', *Early Years Educator*, 8 (3), July: 23–5.

Wyness, M. (2006) *Childhood and Society: An Introduction to the Sociology of Childhood*, Basingstoke: Palgrave Macmillan.

3.2 The child and protection

Not seen, not heard

Lynne Kendall

> There are thousands of different and conflicting definitions of 'child abuse' and 'child neglect' in use today. Definitions have legal, social work, medical, psychological or sociological orientations. Some describe child maltreatment in terms of proscribed parental conduct; some focus on the harm to the child: and many are couched in terms of both. While many definitions share common approaches, elements and even phraseology, the different combinations and permutations seem endless.
>
> (Besharov 1981: 384)

Child abuse is not a relatively new phenomenon. As we look back on the treatment of children throughout history, there have always been adults and parents who have been protective of children and those who have been abusive. Abuse can take many forms and can occur within many settings, including the home environment, institutions, and various education settings. With the advances in modern technology, children and young people can even be abused electronically via text messaging, internet and social networking sites.

This chapter will consider some of the high-profile child abuse cases, the government responses to the subsequent public enquiries and the effectiveness of CRB checks.

There is the notion that child abuse is carried out by strangers, people unknown to the child. Certainly incidents such as the murder of James Bulger and the Dunblane massacre highlight the actions of complete strangers and the consequences of those actions (Hill and Tisdall 1997). Lawrence (2004) argues that there is a widening range of people who may be considered responsible for abuse, from primary caregivers to strangers. However, most abuse is carried out by a person or persons known to the child and often within the home setting, although this is not exclusive. As Hill and Tisdall (1997: 197) acknowledge, 'Revelations by children and adults have shown that suffering "at the hands" of close family members is much more wide spread than had been generally thought'.

Prior to 1988, national statistics on the extent of child abuse were not kept in Britain. However, since 1988 figures have been made available from the Department of Health (Corby 2000). Statistics from the Home Office for child abuse resulting in death in 2007–8 state that there were 69 victims under the age of 16 years (Povey, *et al.* 2009). Forty-three of the victims (62 per cent) were killed by parents, which is an increase of 11 per cent from the years 2006–7. A further 12 (17 per cent) knew the main suspect and 10 (14 per cent) of victims were killed by strangers, as of 4 November 2008. However, these figures do not include deaths by neglect and therefore may not give an accurate figure for the numbers of children who die at the hands of their parents or carers. Figures have not been included for children who are systematically abused but have not died as a result of this abuse.

Historically, if we examine the high-profile deaths of children that have prompted enquiries, each case has similarities. In 1944, Dennis O'Neill, aged 12 years, was in the care of the local authority but was beaten and starved to death by his foster father. The death of Dennis prompted an inquiry in 1945 and the findings of the *Curtis Report* (1946) led to the setting up of the Committee on the Care of Children which later contributed to the Children Act 1948. Maria Colwell, aged seven years, died in 1973 despite 50 official visits to her family acting on complaints made by neighbours to the NSPCC (National Society for the Prevention of Cruelty to Children).

Consider the high-profile cases below:

- Jasmine Beckford (1980)
- Tyra Henry (1984)
- Leanne White (1992)
- Chelsea Brown (1999)
- Lauren Wright (2000).

Each one of these children died as a result of being systematically beaten and abused physically and mentally over a period of time by someone they knew. This was conducted by both parents, an individual parent, step-father or step-mother. The majority of these young children were known to social services, police, health visitors and/or housing officers. Some of the children were in the care of the local authority.

Following the tragic death of each of these children, and many more not listed, there was an inquiry, each one finding failure of all involved to act on warning signs. Since the Children Act 1948 there have been more than 70 inquiries.

The public inquiry in 2003 chaired by Lord Laming, former Chief Inspector of Social Services, into the death of eight-year-old Victoria Climbié, who died as a result of abuse in 2000, highlighted many failings in the child protection system (Lord Laming 2003). Victoria was a child in the care of her great aunt who was fostering her as a private arrangement between herself and Victoria's parents. She was systematically beaten and abused by her great aunt and her great aunt's boyfriend over a prolonged period of time. Despite being in regular contact with four local authorities, two police protection teams, two hospitals, and social workers, Victoria's abuse went unnoticed. There were 12 missed opportunities for professionals to act on what they saw. Examination after Victoria's death revealed 128 separate injuries. The findings from the inquiry identified a failure to protect this child by social workers, police, doctors, NSPCC, and others. There was a failure to share information, lack of effective training, poor management and poor co-ordination between the differing services.

Historically, the findings of each inquiry have fed into national or local policies in the hope that there will not be a repeat of history. The government's response to Lord Laming's inquiry was the Green Paper, *Every Child Matters* (2003). There were four key themes that included: supporting families and carers; ensuring early intervention; addressing issues such as accountability; and ensuring that all people who work with children are trained with the emphasis on collaboration between differing agencies. As Lord Laming stated within the Victoria Climbié inquiry:

It is the hope of the full inquiry team that the horror of what happened to Victoria will endure as a reproach to bad practice and be a beacon pointing the way to securing the safety and well-being of all children in our society.

(2003: 1.68)

Following consultation, the government also passed the Children Act 2004 with *Every Child Matters: Change for Children* being published in November 2004. These new policies were to ensure that in future, children would be safer than ever before.

One could assume that following such a high-profile case, subsequent recommendations and the implementation of the recommendations would result in a decline in incidents of child abuse. In 2005, Deraye Lewis, aged three years, died at the hands of his mother's boyfriend. In 2006, the document *Working Together to Safeguard Children: A Guide to Inter-agency Working to Safeguard and Promote the Welfare of Children* (DfES 2006) was published, with the aim of setting out how the differing organizations can work together effectively.

In 2007, Leticia Wright, who was four years of age, died from abuse by her mother and her boyfriend, a month after a visit by social workers. Neighbours had alerted the council but the file was closed. Another high-profile case was that of 'Baby P', killed in 2007 (following the conviction of Baby P's step-father in 2009, the child was identified as Peter). Social workers, health visitors, police and doctors saw the child 60 times in the eight months leading to his death, with one doctor failing to notice that the child had a broken back. The response to this tragic death was again a public inquiry chaired by Lord Laming. In March 2009 the review published 58 recommendations as part of an action plan to be implemented in April 2009. Among the recommendations was the call for the overhaul of the training and management of children's social workers. Again, as with previous inquires, the same areas in need of improvement have been highlighted and identified. These include the need for better inter-agency working, communication of all involved and better recording, supervision and management. Interestingly the recommendation by Lord Laming that there should be a better recording system is an issue also raised by social workers, who argue that the amount of paper work to be completed prevents them from being in the field. In an article published in the *Independent* (Lakhani 2008), one social worker claimed that 70 per cent of her work involves paperwork and in order to complete this, she spends three evenings and her lunchtimes on this task each week. Research conducted by Harlow and Shardlow (2006) suggests that complete openness and sharing of information with colleagues is not always possible and there are many inhibitors to the development of positive inter-professional relationships which include recruitment and retaining of social workers as well as 'the emotionally distressing and risky nature of safeguarding children' (71).

Consider the following statement taken from the Victoria Climbié Inquiry in 2003:

> Improvements to the way information is exchanged within and between agencies are imperative if children are to be adequately safeguarded.

(Lord Laming 2003: 19: 1.43)

An independent report published in April 2009 into the death of 'Baby Jack', aged six months, highlighted failings in the sharing of information by Tameside Social Services. This child was not on the child protection register, but had been visited on four occasions by a health visitor who failed to gain access to the child. This should have alerted the services and appropriate action should have then been taken. Failings were also attributed to the hospital where the child was taken. Although seriously ill and underweight, the hospital discharged him back into the care of his parents. He died in November 2006 and his parents were subsequently jailed following trial for child cruelty. Again, this child's death was preventable.

DfES (2006) clearly states that if a child is suspected of being at risk of harm, then there is a requirement for all agencies (for example, the local authority, police, children's social care) to meet for the purpose of a strategy discussion that determines whether section 47 of the 1989 Children Act, whereby a child who is suspected of being at risk of serious harm is removed from the situation and placed in care, should be implemented.

Each time a child's death makes the headlines in the media, there is an inquiry into what went wrong. Where did procedures go wrong? When did management of the cases break down? Why was multi-agency working ineffective? And how can the deaths of young children be prevented in the future? Collaborative work between agencies is essential. Many of the child-death inquiry reports have shown that in part, it has been the failure or breakdown of collaborative working or communication that has contributed to the death of a child (Wilson and James 2002).

Wilson and James (2002: 53) suggest that 'There is a need to recognise the fact that it is not the "procedures" but parents' social circumstances, attitudes and behaviour that need to be changed in order to prevent children being impetuously attacked'.

Activity 3.2.1: The effectiveness of public inquiries

Having read the above, consider and discuss the following questions:

- How effective are public inquiries?
- What do they achieve?
- What factors may contribute to child abuse within the family?

Defining child abuse

There are many definitions of what constitutes child abuse. Lawrence (2004: 8) suggests that these definitions are 'fraught with both cultural and value based difficulties' and Corby (2000: 66) acknowledges that 'Child abuse is a socially defined construct. It is the product of a particular culture and context and not an absolute unchanging phenomenon'.

Definitions of what constitutes child abuse are also dependent upon what one believes is an acceptable or unacceptable way of treating children within differing social groups (Munro 2002: 61) Munro also suggests that there is a difficulty in defining abuse precisely, so that there can be an agreement by all concerned as to which actions are abusive and how serious these actions are.

However, in a simplistic form, abuse can be described as an action by an adult that causes either physical harm, psychological harm, or both to a child. In her definition of child abuse, Munro (2002) not only talks about abuse being a way of treating a child that is harmful but also suggests that it is 'morally' wrong as well.

The NSPCC suggests that child abuse can take four forms which are recognized as the standard four sub-categories of abuse, however, there are other terms that are also used to describe behaviours which can cause harm to children. Below are definitions of the different types of abuse.

Physical abuse: This includes hitting, shaking, kicking, punching and other forms of inflicting pain or an injury to a child. This may also include giving a child any harmful substance such as alcohol, poison or other types of drugs (NSPCC).

The definition of physical abuse in DfES (2006) also states that 'Physical harm may also be caused when a parent or carer feigns the symptoms of, or deliberately causes ill health to a child (8). This is often referred to as Munchhausen's syndrome by proxy (MSBP). Beckett (2007: 66) discusses issues surrounding MSBP and the ways that the child protection system can get it wrong with mothers being accused of killing their own children, having other children removed from them and being sent to prison.

Emotional abuse: This is when behaviours by a parent or a carer are likely to affect a child's emotional development which are often difficult to identify. This abuse can be via constant rejection, withdrawal of affection, humiliation and constant criticism (NSPCC).

All children are subjected to emotional abuse to some degree, take for example, the adult who has said or done something unkind in anger, immediately regretting what they have said or done (Beckett 2007: 71). However, in DfES (2006) part of the definition of emotional abuse is the emphasis on 'the *persistent* emotional maltreatment of a child'. The document also acknowledges that the over protection of children can also be considered emotional abuse (39).

Emotional abuse cannot be physically seen and for intervention purposes it can be extremely difficulty to pinpoint, however the consequences of such actions can have a lifelong impact upon a child. It is also important to consider that all abuse involves some emotional ill treatment (Wilson and James 2002) and the Department of Health (2000) guidelines suggest that while emotional abuse can occur by itself (supported by DfES 2006: 1: 31) it is certainly more likely to accompany, or be the consequence of, other forms of abuse (Corby 2000).

Neglect: Defined as a lack of appropriate care, which includes love, safety, nourishment, warmth, medical attention, education. Such a lack can impact upon a child's physical, mental and emotional development (NSPCC). The definition of neglect in DfES (2006) emphasizes that neglect can occur during pregnancy as a result of maternal substance abuse such as alcohol abuse, which can result in the child having foetal alcohol syndrome, or the abuse of other drugs.

Beckett (2007: 69) suggests that the definitions given of emotional abuse and neglect within DfES (2006) overlap and indeed 'shade into each other' and it is often difficult to distinguish these two areas.

Sexual abuse: Defined as pressurizing, tricking or forcing a child or young person into taking part in any kind of sexual activity. This can also include encouraging a child to look at pornographic materials (NSPCC). Statistics show that the sexual abuser is often known to the child. Of the 13,237 children counselled for sexual abuse by ChildLine in 2007–8, the vast majority were abused by someone they knew: 59 per cent said that they had been sexually abused by a family member; 29 per cent said they had been sexually abused by someone else known to them; and 4 per cent said they had been sexually abused by a stranger (statistics released by the NSPCC in 2009).

Beckett (2007) considers that sexual abuse does not always manifest itself in a physical way but certainly there would be signs and symptoms that may manifest in behavioural issues that may indicate the possibility of sexual abuse.

The NSPCC further acknowledge that bullying and domestic violence can impact upon a child/young person with serious consequences.

There is the assumption that families are often the best environment in which to raise children, which is often far from the truth. McKie (2005: 31) suggests that cultural attitudes and assumptions also play a part in the reporting of violence to the relevant authorities and families may not report violence because of a sense of shame and the associated taboos surrounding violence within families.

There are other forms of child mistreatment to be considered, such as child prostitution, ritual abuse (consider the Orkney case in 1991), domestic violence, bullying (Beckett 2007; Corby 2000) and the impact that mental health issues concerning a parent/carer may have upon a child. An extreme example is that of Jael Mullings, a young mother who killed her two young children in November 2008 and was consequently detained under the Mental Health Act. The family were known to social services but the children were not on the at-risk register.

It is important to be aware of the overlap of each of these categories. They may not stand in isolation; if a child experiences physical abuse or sexual abuse, this is often accompanied by emotional abuse (Wilson and James 2002).

Cross-cultural considerations

The actions of child abuse are certainly not clearly defined across differing cultures in society and what is considered acceptable by one culture may be viewed as abusive practice by another (Corby 2000; Munro 2002). An example of this is female foeticide, the killing of a female child in the womb, and female infanticide. In some countries such as India, there is a cultural preference for sons (Munro 2002). A girl may be seen as a financial liability, particularly in relation to costly dowries when the daughter marries. The practice of female foeticide is not permitted under Indian Government law, however this practice continues (Bryant 2007).

Female foeticide is not confined to the poor either; increased wealth also brings access to prenatal ultrasounds and sonograms and the results of such tests allow for termination of a female foetus (Bryant 2007). This alters the sex ratio of boys to girls, as discussed by Dubuc and Coleman (2007).

Consider also the practice of female genital mutilation/cutting, a common practice in West Africa, East Africa and parts of the Middle East. Reports from Europe, North America and Australia suggest that this practice is also carried out among immigrant communities (UNICEF 2005). Under the Female Circumcision Act 1985 and the Female Genital Mutilation Act 2003, this is an illegal practice within the United Kingdom.

Indeed, as Beckett (2007) acknowledges, child protection professionals themselves will come from differing cultural and socio-economic backgrounds, working with a diverse range of clients from not only different cultures but also from differing social classes and with a range of parenting practices and attitudes to childrearing.

Following the tragic death of Victoria Climbié, the report of findings by Lord Laming (2003) suggested that the requirement to keep children safe transcends cultural boundaries and while cultural heritage is important to many people, 'it cannot take precedence over standards of childcare embodied in law' (346: 16: 10) In other words, every child is entitled to protection from the law of this country.

The government has introduced a number of measures to protect children and vulnerable adults, including the creation of the Criminal Records Bureau.

Criminal records check

The murders of the two schoolgirls Holly Wells and Jessica Chapman in Soham, in August 2002 by Ian Huntley highlighted serious flaws in the record system of the Humberside police. Despite Huntley's being known to the police, and having been accused of several sex-related crimes over a number of years, Humberside and Cambridge police failed to spot the allegations during the vetting process that enabled Huntley to be employed as a caretaker at Soham Village College. Records of Huntley's past had been lost and a check had been conducted with the wrong birth-date details and only on the alias that Huntley used. A public inquiry report on child protection procedures was commissioned by the then Home Secretary, David Blunkett.

The Bichard Inquiry Report (Bichard 2004) identified numerous errors in the vetting process:

> The enquiry did find errors, omissions, failures and shortcomings which are deeply shocking. Taken together, these were so extensive that one cannot be confident that it was Huntley alone who slipped through the net.
>
> (1: 6)

Following *The Bichard Inquiry Report*, a number of recommendations were made. These have implications for those working with children and young people in education settings. According to the report, there needs to be a registration scheme for everyone who works with children or vulnerable adults which employers can access. This would show if there was a reason why someone should not work with children. All applications for positions in schools should be subject to a requirement for enhanced-disclosure criminal checks. Training is a necessity for head teachers and school governors to ensure interview panels are aware of the importance of safeguarding children.

The creation of the Criminal Records Bureau (CRB) in 2002 provides criminal record checks on those people who wish to work with children or vulnerable adults. CRB checks are now mandatory for schools, the care home sector and the domiciliary care sector. The CRB can make two types of disclosure about a person's background. The first of these is the standard disclosure, for people who wish to apply for positions that would involve them being in regular contact with young people/children under the age of 18 years. This standard disclosure can be provided for people who are in occupations that involve positions of trust and reveals details of all convictions that have been held on the central police records, including spent convictions. The second type of disclosure is the enhanced disclosure which is required for posts that would involve a far greater degree of contact with children. The enhanced disclosure contains all the same information that is given in a standard disclosure but it also contains any information that is held by the local police.

However, the CRB check is only able to identify that a person may be unsuitable to work with children and vulnerable adults if they already have a criminal record or are on the sex offenders register. The CRB is a 'snapshot in time'. It does not identify any person who may have 'evil intentions or thoughts' towards children and can only give evidence of what has happened in the past, not what may happen in the future. There are loopholes in the system. Take for example the case of Reverend Richard Hart, a vicar in the Anglican Church, who was found guilty in 2008 of taking and possessing sexual images of children. Hart had a CRB check prior to his ordination and also in his capacity as the governor of a local school, however, because he did not have a criminal history he was allowed to work with children. Consider also the issue of people who are falsely accused of wrong doing by the CRB. In the year up to February 2008, 680 people were issued with incorrect information on their background checks (Hope 2008). Consider the case of John Pinnington, who worked with children with learning disabilities. He was sacked from his job when a CRB check revealed that he had been accused of sexually abusing children in his care. These were unfounded accusations which did not result in him being charged. The accusations had been made by an intermediary who had interpreted what the child with learning disabilities had said. Accusations had been passed on to the CRB without any evidence to support them.

From October 2009, any person who is in paid work or works in a voluntary capacity with either children and young people under 18 years of age or vulnerable adults will have to register with the Independent Safeguarding Authority (ISA). The ISA scheme (introduced in light of the Soham murders) requires that anyone who wishes to work with children or vulnerable adults have their backgrounds checked; unregistered persons will not be employed. Checks will be made with the CRB by the ISA workforce and this should ensure that the person to be employed is suitable to work within certain settings. Following on from the ruling in the case of John Pinnington, this new system will allow accusations to be retained and passed on, remaining on the database, even if there is no evidence to support them.

However, an article written in the *Telegraph* in January 2009 highlights that there are limitations to the new vetting setting, with loopholes in the vetting procedure (Beckford 2009). The CRB is unable to check if applicants have been found guilty of crimes in most overseas countries. Most crimes that have been committed by immigrants in their home countries or by British nationals abroad (including paedophile convictions) will not be recorded. Gaining access to criminal records from foreign governments is proving difficult. To date, only three of the 26 European Union countries have agreed to exchange files for vetting. Surprisingly, there will be no requirement for the ISA to check if applicants have lived or worked abroad. As Bichard (2004) notes:

> For those agencies whose job it is to protect children and vulnerable people, the harsh reality is that if a sufficiently devious person is determined to seek out opportunities to work their evil, no one can guarantee that they will be stopped. Our task is to make it as difficult as possible for them to succeed.
>
> (12: 79)

Activity 3.2.2: Loopholes in vetting systems

Consider the following:

- What 'problems' do loopholes in vetting procedures pose for employers?
- What are the implications of these loopholes for children and vulnerable people in education, health and social care?

Conclusion

This chapter has highlighted government responses, both historical and contemporary, to cases of child abuse that have resulted in the tragic deaths of so many children. Each inquiry considers what should have been done, the various contributive failings, apportions blame to the agencies involved and makes recommendations for future practice. The question has to be asked: Can the abuse of children and young people ever be totally prevented? Perhaps we need to consider how many more Victoria Climbiés or Baby Ps would there have been if these enquiries had not taken place. As yet, it is too soon to consider how effective the recommendations made by Lord Laming following the death of Baby P will be.

Student reflection

The NSPCC and the current government have called for a 'full stop' to child abuse.

• Do you think child abuse can ever be completely eradicated?

Key points

• There are difficulties in defining child abuse.
• Abuse can take many forms, including physical, emotional, neglect and sexual, and these can overlap.
• Parents, and other adults known to the child, are responsible for the vast majority of cases of child abuse, including those which result in the death of the child.
• A number of inquiries into the death of children from child abuse express the need for more effective inter-agency information sharing.
• The CRB was established to help safeguard children but it is not failsafe and only provides information on those who have already offended.
• There are issues with information stored by the CRB and ISA in that unproven allegations may be recorded.

Recommended reading

Cullingford, C. (2007) *Childhood – The Inside Story: Hearing Children's Voices*, Newcastle: Cambridge.
Dale, Peter, Green, Richard and Fellows, Ron (2005) *Child Protection Assessment Following Serious Injuries to Infants: Fine Judgments*, Chichester: John Wiley & Sons Ltd.
Jenks, Chris (2005) *Childhood*, 2nd edn, Abingdon: Routledge.
Jones, Liz, Holmes, Rachel and Powell, John (eds) (2005) *Early Childhood Studies: A Multiprofessional Approach*, Maidenhead: McGraw-Hill/OUP.

References

Beckett, Chris (2007) *Child Protection: An Introduction*, 2nd edn, London: Sage Publications Ltd.
Beckford, Martin (2009) 'Foreign criminals could work in English schools under "major loophole"', *Daily Telegraph*, 1 January.
Besharov, Douglas (1981) 'Towards better research on child abuse and neglect: making definitional

issues an explicit methodological concern', *Child Abuse and Neglect: The International Journal*, 5 (4): 383–90.

Bichard, M (2004) *The Bichard Inquiry Report*, London: HMSO.

Bryant, Nick (2007) 'Girls at risk amid India's prosperity', BBC News. Available online at: http://news.bbc.co.uk/1/hi/world/south_asia/6934540.stm (accessed 2 April 2009).

Corby, Brian (2000) *Child Abuse: Towards a Knowledge Base*, 2nd edn, Berkshire: Open University Press.

Curtis Report (1946) *Report of the Care of Children Committee*, London: HMSO.

DfES (Department for Education and Skills) (2006) *Working Together to Safeguard Children: a Guide to Inter-agency Working to Safeguard and Promote the Welfare of Children*. London: The Stationery Office.

Dubuc, Sylvie and Coleman, David (2007) 'An increase in the sex ratio of births to India-born mothers in England and Wales: evidence for sex-selection abortion', *Population and Development Review*, 33 (2): 383–400.

Harlow, Elizabeth and Shardlow, Steven, M. (2006) 'Safeguarding children: challenges to the effective operation of core groups, *Child and Family Social Work*, 11: 65–72.

Hill, Malcolm and Tisdall, Kay (1997) *Children and Society*, Essex: Pearson Education Limited.

Hope, Christopher (2008) 'Hundreds of innocent people "wrongly branded criminals" by CRB checks', *Daily Telegraph*, 5 July.

Lakhani, Nina (2008) 'Social workers: on the frontline', *Independent*, 16 November.

Lawrence, Anne (2004) *Principles of Child Protection: Management and Practice*, Berkshire: Open University Press.

Lord Laming (2003) *The Victoria Climbié Inquiry*, London: HMSO.

—— (2009) *The Protection of Children in England: A Progress Report*, London: The Stationery Office.

McKie, Linda (2005) *Families, Violence and Social Change*, Berkshire: Open University Press.

Munro, Eileen (2002) *Effective Child Protection*, London: Sage Publications Ltd.

NSPCC (National Society for the Prevention of Cruelty to Children) (2009) 'Children counselled for sexual abuse by ChildLine reaches new high', Press Release, 9 February. Available online at: http://www.nspcc.org.uk/whatwedo/mediacentre/pressreleases/2009_09_february_children_counselled_for_sexual_abuse_by_ChildLine_reaches_new_high_wdn63429.html (accessed 2 April 2009).

Povey, David (ed.), Coleman, Kathryn, Kaiza, Peter, Roe, Stephen (2009) *Homicides, Firearm Offences and Intimate Violence 2007/08 (Supplementary Volume 2 to Crime in England and Wales 2007/08)*. Home Office Statistical Bulletin 02/09.

UNICEF (2005) *Female Genital Mutilation/Cutting: A Statistical Exploration*, New York: UNICEF.

Wilson, Kate and James, Adrian (2002) *The Child Protection Handbook*, 2nd edn, Edinburgh, London and New York: Bailliere Tindall.

3.3 Life as a looked-after child
The parent of last resort

Derek Kassem

There are approximately 70,000 children (DCSF 2008a; Welsh Assembly Government 2008; The Scottish Government 2008) who are in the care of the state within the UK and they are formally referred to as 'looked-after children'. Looked-after children is a term that was first used in the 1989 Children Act and subsequent Acts in the various jurisdictions that make up the legal system within the UK. This comparatively small number represents a tiny percentage of the 13.1 million children under the age of 18 who live in the UK. Yet with the state as their parent, the life chances and experience of being in the care system can only be desribed as appalling for substantial numbers of looked-after children. It should be noted that not all looked-after children suffer the outcomes described below. The challenges that looked-after children face are extensive. Firstly, the experiences leading up to and entering the care system are often traumatic for the child. For many children the experiences of the care system can be just as traumatic as their experiences before entering the system, if not more so. The final challenge is the attitude towards looked-after children by the wider society. All these elements come together to create a childhood that some individuals find almost impossible to overcome, with the resultant poor life chances.

The parent of last resort

Children enter the care system primarily because they are in need of care and protection. The specific reasons a child might enter the care system are varied and include abuse in a variety of forms such as neglect, sexual, physical and emotional, or in some cases a combination of all of these forms. Abuse is not the only reason a child may be taken into care; another cause could be a breakdown in the family. This may be due to a major crisis varying from the death of a parent to parental drug and alcohol addiction. Asylum-seeking children travelling alone or trafficked children are also deemed to be looked-after children as a result of a combination of the Children Act (1989) and a number of court judgments. Very young children, namely babies, can enter the care system as a result of unwanted pregnancies and are usually put up for adoption. However, some babies are removed from the mother at birth. This may be due to previous concerns regarding the parents' behaviours in respect of their ability to care for the child. Only a small percentage of children are taken into the care system because of their criminal activities. Yet the view that looked-after status is somehow linked to criminality is a challenge that looked-after children face, for as one young care leaver states:

As soon as you say you are in care, people stigmatise. Some people seem to think that a child is in care because they have done something wrong.

Kate Morris – Manchester Metropolitan University graduate who went into care at the age of nine. (*Times Educational Supplement* 23 December 2005)

It should be remembered that looked-after children have the state for a parent because they are in need of care and protection. Kate Morris's view of how looked-after children are perceived by the general public is not in any way exaggerated or unique to her. A survey carried out by A National Voice, the main organization for looked-after children run by looked-after children, found that only 8 per cent of children in care felt that the general public viewed them as the same as other young people (A National Voice 2002). The survey also found that 20 per cent of the children involved in the study thought the public viewed them as 'untrustworthy', 25 per cent felt they were seen as trouble makers and 13 per cent thought that the general public saw them in need of sympathy (ibid.). The stereotypes used as shorthand to deal with looked-after children impact on the lives of the child in all areas of their lives, not least education. These attitudes to children in care are just one of the factors that play a role in their life chances.

Looked-after children: the outcomes

The results of being in care, with the state as a parent, are extremely bleak. The *Guardian* (Gentleman 2009) reported that 53 per cent of looked-after children left school with no General Certificates of Secondary Education (GCSEs); only 13 per cent achieved five A*–C grade GCSEs, compared to 47 per cent for the age group as a whole. Only 6 per cent of looked-after children manage to get to university, while 29 per cent are not in any form of education, employment or training by the age of 19. However, it is not just the individual children who pay a price for the increase in social exclusion and the failure of the state as a parent – it is also the wider society as a whole. For the educational outcomes are not the only factors that display failure on the part of the state to provide a better life for looked-after children. For instance, 20 per cent of women who leave care between the ages of 16 and 19 become mothers within a year of leaving care. In other words, looked-after girls are two and a half times more likely to become teenage parents (SEU 1999). Roughly a quarter (23 per cent) of the prison population has been through the care system (SEU 2002). The percentage in prison should also be placed in the context of an ever increasing prison population. In terms of youth offenders, 30 per cent of young offenders have also been through the care system and finally 45 per cent of looked-after children have been assessed as having a mental health disorder.

Looked-after children are also a significant presence among the most socially deprived members of our society. For instance, between 25 per cent and a third of rough sleepers were in care (SEU 2003). This figure is similar to the one identified by the *Big Issue* who found around 18 per cent of their vendors had been in care at sometime in their lives (*Big Issue* 2001). One of the most distressing outcomes for looked-after children is identified by a Home Office study into vulnerable people (Cusick, Martin and May 2003) which found that 42 per cent of the sex workers interviewed had spent some period of their childhood being looked after. The same study also found similar rates for drug users. This is not to say of course that all children who have been through the care system have unsuccessful lives – quite the contrary – but a great many do have problems due to their life experiences.

Activity 3.3.1: How the UK system for looked-after children compares

- Research the way looked-after children are cared for in Denmark and/or Germany.
- What are the main differences between the Danish and German systems, and the system in the UK?

All of these outcomes impact on society as a whole. The failure of the state as a parent not only impacts on the individual child in care but on the wider society as well. Society inevitably pays a price, for example, the costs associated with an ever growing prison population and the costs associated with drug addiction and homelessness, all of which are outcomes for an unacceptable number of looked-after children from their teenage years to adulthood. The failure of the care system is in many respects unique to the UK as our European neighbours such as Germany, Denmark or similar industrialized countries do not match it (Petrie, *et al.* 2006 and Kassem 2009). Such are the poor outcomes for the UK's looked-after children that even relatively poor European powers such as Portugal have had better results in supporting their looked-after children. The UK is at the bottom of the league table for the quality of outcomes of the care system (Petrie, *et al.* 2006). The argument that the state is failing the very children that it claims to be providing care and protection for is indisputable. To understand this failure, it is necessary to recognize the social factors that lead up to a child entering the care system and the problems within the care system itself.

That a child is in need of care and protection is as much a product of the individuals in that child's life as the socio-economic circumstances in which the family exists. The impact of poverty on families and the link between poverty and child abuse is a largely ignored aspect of the child protection system. The focus is on the individuals rather than the context in which they exist. In part, this adds to the problems that the child protection and care system face in supporting children and families.

Poverty

Child poverty has been substantially on the increase since 1979:

> After 1979, with rapidly growing inequality (and with some growth in numbers of children in groups, particularly lone parents, which have traditionally been poor), many families with children were left behind as societal income rose, thus explaining the rapid rise in child poverty. This increase levelled off in the 1990s but did not fall until after 1998. In the last two years of data, child poverty has risen.
>
> (Child Poverty Action Group 2008: 7)

As indicated above, poverty rates in the UK have been substantially higher over the last 30 years than they were in the 1960s and 70s. To understand the impact of poverty on the child, it is necessary to recognize the multidimensional nature of poverty and the way it affects different members of family units. The impact of poverty on children is not the same as the impact of poverty on parents (Magadi and Middleton 2007; Ferguson and Lavalette 2009). Child poverty has many long-term implications for the individual, not least in their health and well-being (Hirsch 2007). The behaviours that some looked-after children display, such as disaffection, resentment and low academic achievement are also strongly associated with child deprivation. The commonality of behaviours exhibited by some children in poverty and looked-after children should not be considered surprising if the relationship between children on the at-risk register and poverty is recognized, for children on the at-risk register are all potentially looked-after children.

The relationship between geographical location of areas of poverty and relatively high levels of potential child abuse can only be described as startling. One study found that 60 per cent of children on the at-risk register in Strathclyde in the 1990s were from Glasgow, which has the highest concentration of poverty but only 27 per cent of the region's population (Baldwin and Spencer 1993). The highest concentration of children at risk in Glasgow was to be found in the three poorest areas. In a study of a different city, approximately 25 per cent of children on the child protection register in the City of Coventry lived within the poorest ward of the city though it held only 12 per cent of the city's children (Baldwin and Carruthers 1998). This relationship between poverty and child abuse should be seen against the backdrop of the growth of income inequality which is now at a 40-year high – not since the early 1960s has the gap between the richest and poorest been so great (Brewer, *et al.* 2009). It is therefore no surprise that social deprivation rose for a third successive year in 2007–8, with the income of the poorest in society showing a marked decline in their living standards (ibid.). Devaney (2009) has linked the extent of social deprivation through key markers such as unemployment, dependence on state benefits and poor housing to a positive relationship with children being placed on the child protection register. Although this chapter is not about child protection but rather looked-after children, the process of entering the care system often starts with concerns around child protection. Child protection is clearly linked to children being taken into the care system and just as poverty is a key factor in child protection, poverty is also a major factor in whether a child enters the care system (Statham, *et al.* 2002). Of course not all poor parents or children face the problems that result in the child entering the care system, though there is a link between poverty and child protection issues.

Activity 3.3.2: Consequences of childhood poverty

- How does poverty in childhood impact on the child as an adult?
- Research the relationship between child poverty and adult health outcomes.

Mental health

Mental health concerns among young people who are looked-after are dramatic in the extent to which they exist compared to the general population of the same age group. Forty-five per cent of children aged between five and 17 years of age who are in the care system have been identified as having a mental disorder of some kind (National Statistics 2003). Of these:

> Thirty seven per cent had clinically significant conduct disorders; twelve per cent were assessed as having emotional disorders – anxiety and depression – and seven per cent were rated as hyperactive

> (National Statistics 2003)

In the same study, the National Statistics Office provided direct comparisons of mental health issues between looked-after children and a representative sample of 10,500 children living in private households. Table 3.3.1 clearly indicates the massive differences between the two groups of children.

The mental health picture of very young children who are looked-after is fundamentally different from that of their peers who live outside the care system. The mental health of their older brothers and sisters does not show any improvement except in one area – that of hyperkinetic disorders. Apart from this one category, as indicated below, the mental health of the children shows a marked deterioration.

The data below only give part of the story of the mental health of looked-after children who live in residential care. Children living in residential care, normally referred to as a children's home, show a greater degree of what can only be desribed as distress, as 68 per cent of children living in residential care exhibited or were assessed as having a mental disorder, while 39 per cent of children living in foster care and 42 per cent living with their birth parents were assessed as having a mental disorder (National Statistics 2003). Clearly, those children in residential care can be said to be suffering to the greatest degree. Similar outcomes for children in residential care have been found in other studies (e.g. Richardson and Lelliott 2003). Residential care seems to pose some very specific difficulties which are not entirely unique to the UK. Schmid, *et al.* (2008) found that children living in children's homes in Germany were also a neglected high-risk population.

The socio-demographics of residential care demonstrate a marked difference from that of foster or kinship care. One study found that there were nearly twice as many boys in residential care compared to girls (Ford, *et al.* 2007). Residential care is also frequently used for children with the most difficulties and who have had a number of foster

Table 3.3.1 Prevalence of mental disorders among 5- to 10-year-olds (%)

Condition	Looked-after children	Children living in private households
Emotional disorders	11	3
Conduct disorders	36	5
Hyperkinetic disorders	11	2
Any childhood disorder	42	8

Source: National Statistics (2003).

Table 3.3.2 Prevalence of mental disorders among 11- to 15-year-olds (%)

Condition	Looked-after children	Children living in private households
Emotional disorders	12	6
Conduct disorders	40	6
Hyperkinetic disorders	7	1
Any childhood disorder	49	11

Source: National Statistics (2003).

placements fail. Children who live in residential care tend to be concentrated around the older age bracket and therefore find it harder to find foster placements and adoption is a very remote possibility. This study also showed that apart from being in residential care, another major factor in the mental health of looked-after children was placement instability (ibid.). Richarson and Lelliott (2003) suggest that the social disadvantage and poverty experienced by looked-after children prior to entry into the care system is accentuated by the care system itself. The frequent changing of accommodation creates stress and insecurity in the child. It should also be pointed out that there is a regular turnover of staff in residential children's homes, which in part is due to the low pay and very low level of qualifications and training experienced by residential social workers in the UK (Petrie, *et al.* 2006; Kassem 2009). It should be noted that an individual does not need any qualifications to work in a children's home. The government target to remedy this lack of professional education is for residential social workers to achieve level 3 of the National Vocational Qualification. In comparison, Denmark requires all residential social workers to be educated to degree level with appropriate training (Petrie, *et al.* 2006). The subsequent quality of care is far higher and the children in residential care in Denmark exhibited much lower levels of the worst outcomes that looked-after children do in the UK. In fact, looked-after children in Denmark achieve a great deal more success than in the UK. This is even more startling when the majority of looked-after children in Denmark live in residential care, while in the UK only 11 per cent of looked-after children do (Petrie, *et al.* 2006). The level of qualification is indicative of the investment and quality of resources that are given over to looked-after children in Denmark compared to the UK.

Residential care often has a poor record for mental health outcomes for looked-after children and this needs to be addressed, however, it would be a mistake to think that foster care or kinship placements were fundamentally different in outcomes. All looked-after children, no matter the nature of the placement and care provisions provided, suffer from higher levels of mental disorders compared to their peers in the general population. Not only does the care system fail to address the issues that looked-after children faced prior to entry into the care system, in many respects, it also accentuates them. Insecurity, movement from one place to another and the concomitant changes of schools are all experienced by children living in poverty – the care system then all too often repeats the experience again.

Activity 3.3.3: Looked-after children and mental disorders

- Reflect on why looked-after children suffer from such high levels of mental disorders compared to their peers.
- What do you think could be done to help looked-after children in distress?

Education

Educational outcomes have improved over the last few years, with looked-after children making progress to achieving similar levels as their peers (DCSF 2008b). However, this small positive does not capture the full picture regarding education of looked-after children because, as indicated above, the level of attainment is still low. For instance, only a small percentage of looked-after children gain a university place (DCSF 2008b). Too many looked-after children are failed by the education system in all the benchmarks used by the government to identify levels of academic attainment in the wider community. As with mental health needs, looked-after children have some very specific educational needs that are not addressed by schools, such as special needs, bullying support and literacy and numeracy difficulties.

Looked-after children have been identified as being at least a year behind their peers in their intellectual development (National Statistics 2003). Approximately 27 per cent of looked-after children are also identified as having a special educational need (Kassem 2006). A recent parliamentary select committee identified the percentage of children with a special educational need at 28 per cent (House of Commons 2009). Looked-after children are ten times more likely to have a statement of special educational need as their peers. That children in care have educational difficulties should not be a surprise, as children who suffer from high levels of social and economic deprivation also follow a similar pattern (Magadi and Middleton 2007) and, as it has already been argued, there is a strong relationship between poverty and the care system. The similarities across the mental health issues of looked-after children are stark. The very systems that are supposedly put in place to aid and support looked-after children do not function, are ignored or effectively work against the children.

Looked-after children now have the legal right to go to the school of their choice. This legal right was given to looked-after children in an attempt to redress the educational disadvantages they face. However, schools often ignore this right of access to looked-after children. The rejection of children in need by the education system is also common to children in poverty. The Sutton Trust (2006) found that the best-performing comprehensive schools located in poor and economically deprived areas had much lower numbers of children entitled to free school meals than would be expected due to their location. Free school meal entitlement is a recognized but imperfect indicator of child poverty. The new Academies aimed at, according to government policy, the needs of children from deprived backgrounds follow the same pattern as the already established comprehensive schools by reducing the numbers of children on the roll entitled to free school dinners (Wrigley 2009). The rejection by schools of the poor and looked-after children is easy to understand. The schools' success is based on measurable outcomes that are very restricted in form. A school's standing in the community, local authority and in published league tables is determined to a large extent by the number of GCSEs at grade A*–C their pupils achieve or, in the primary sector, the number of level 4s and 5s at the end of Key Stage assessment. Those children who have a special need, be it behavioural or learning, can be seen to be a liability – that is they will not get the grades and at the same time take up more resources.

The rejection of looked-after children is also linked to their greater rates of permanent exclusion from school. Looked-after children have comparatively high levels of school exclusion rates. A child in care is ten times more likely to be excluded from school than their peers. School exclusion clearly impacts on a child's education in a number of ways, not least the missing of school and the resultant change of schools. The exclusion adds to the instability and insecurity that the looked-after child experiences. The school exclusion rates also, in common with the socially deprived, tend to impact on boys more than girls (DCSF 2008c). Boys are four times more likely to be excluded than girls are. It should also be noted that children with a special need are nine times more likely to be excluded from school compared to children without a special need (DCSF 2008c). If one takes into account that the looked-after child is more likely to have a special need and that there are slightly more boys in the care system, then these factors, together with the looked-after status and the mental health concerns, paint a very poor picture for the extent and quality of education that children in care receive.

There are other factors that impact on the education of looked-after children, including low teacher expectations (Kassem 2006) and bullying by peers (Morris 2000) that go to create the poor levels of attainment. What the reader should recognize, however, is that though a bleak picture has been painted, some looked-after children do succeed and achieve high educational standards; they just tend to be in the minority. The lives of looked-after children are not just impacted upon by poverty, mental health disorders and poor education – looked-after children also figure disproportionately in crime figures. Specifically, higher percentages of looked-after children find themselves in young offenders' institutions and, as adults, in prison.

Young offenders

The relationship between offending and care may exist within the mind of the general public but it is far more complex than that simple correlation. What is true, however, is that a child in care over the age of criminal responsibility (ten years in England, this varies across the different jurisdictions in the UK) are three times more likely to be cautioned or convicted of an offence than their peers (Taylor 2006). The Youth Justice Board (Hazel, *et al.* 2002) carried out a study that found 41 per cent of children in youth custody came from a background in the care system. Given that the percentage of children in care is only 0.5 per cent of the total number of children in the UK, these figures can only be described as significant (Department for Health 2003). This cannot be explained through an assumption that looked-after status is linked to criminality because very few children are taken into the care system for criminal behaviour (see above). The numbers of looked-after children must be taken as a wider part of the increased numbers of young people being sentenced to custody. The Prison Reform Trust (2008) found that the number of girls between the ages of ten and 17 sentenced at magistrate's court increased by a staggering 181 per cent over the period 1996–2006. This massive increase in custodial sentences is more a product of policy than any major increase in crime by young women. The increased use of custodial sentences for young people does not apply equally across the country. For example, children have a one in ten chance of being jailed for a non-violent offence in the Home Counties but a one in fifty chance of being jailed for the very same offence in inner-city Newcastle (Verkaik 2009). This suggests that the increase in custodial sentences is more a product of policy rather than an increase in crime or the nature of the offence. The Youth Justice Board has actually stated a custodial sentence is more likely to be applied to a child if the local magistrates lack confidence in the local authority provision of supported accommodation (ibid.). These policy variations, coupled with the political decision to be tough on crime, result in the increase of children being sent to prison often for comparatively minor offences, such as a breach of an Anti-Social Behaviour Order (ASBO).

The background of young offenders reads almost identically to that of looked-after children in many respects: poverty, low self-esteem, poor literacy and numeracy, school exclusion and experience of abuse. Clearly, the limited evidence above indicates that young offenders are some of the most deprived children in the UK. The overlap between looked-after children and young offenders arises, in part, as a consequence of the child entering the care system. In effect, the care system itself contributes to the child's

Table 3.3.3 Some characteristics of children in prison (%)

Percentage of children with previous convictions entering prison (15–17-year-olds)	15
Children in custody who have been involved with, or in the care of, social services before entering custody	71
Children in custody previously homeless	40
Prevalence of mental health problems among children in prison	85
Young women (under 18) who self-harmed in custody	89

Source: Prison Reform Trust (2008).

offending, yet once a child has entered the youth justice system the extent to which their previous experiences of the care system are taken into account is limited.

The irony of the youth offender institutions is that they replicate the experiences that led the child to custody from the care system, for because placement instability is a key issue for the care system the Prison Reform Trust (2008) has identified the high numbers of movements of children around the system to make way for new arrivals, thus disrupting education and training. It would seem not to matter which part of the system a child is in – care or youth offending – the essential experience of the provision remains the same.

Conclusion

This chapter has attempted to identify two main concerns in the life of looked-after children: poverty and what might be called system-wide neglect. The commonalities between the socially deprived, the looked-after, the child with mental health disorders and the young offender all add up. The problems that looked-after children face are rooted in the social inequality that exists within our society which is increasing and will get worse in the light of the economic recession. The inequalities are compounded by the lack of investment in the care system at all levels, in particular pay rates for residential social workers. In part, the low pay is due to the low level of qualifications that is needed to become a residential social worker, which currently stands at life experience and nothing else. Equally, the quality of training, education and support for the foster care system also needs to be improved along with a questioning of the cottage industry approach in foster care that currently seems acceptable. Caring for children to pay off the mortgage is unacceptable. Social workers need a level of investment that allows for a caseload that is workable and where the children can and do develop a relationship with the social worker.

Although there is some very good provision, the scale of the problems for 0.5 per cent of the children in this country is evidence enough that the system does not work. Until a major restructuring and investment in the care system occurs, perhaps on the lines of Denmark (Petrie, *et al.* 2006), the problems will occur generation after generation. Even if fundamental changes are made to the care system, the reality of child poverty will always hinder and obstruct the improvements made in the care system – in other words, child poverty is the greatest form of child abuse that is effectively ignored by society as a whole, except in politicians' political flourishes of high-sounding rhetoric that all too often come to nothing.

Student reflection

• Why do you think that looked-after children are often seen as young criminals in people's minds rather than as children in need of care and protection?

Key points

• Looked-after children are failed by the care system.
• Poverty plays a major role in child protection issues as well as in children entering the care system.
• Looked-after children, for the most part, under-achieve educationally.
• Significant numbers of looked-after children suffer from mental health disorders.
• Significant numbers of looked-after children become criminalized while in the care system.
• Residential care social workers are low paid and poorly qualified.
• Foster carers need more training and support.
• Countries such as Denmark and Germany provide for their looked-after children far more successfully than the UK.

Recommended reading

Hewitt, P. (2002) *The Looked After Kid: My Life in a Children's Home*, Edinburgh: Mainstream Publishing.
Chase, E., *et al.* (eds) (2006) *In Care and After: A Positive Perspective*, London: Routledge.
Petrie, P., Boddy, J., Cameron, C., Wigfall, C. and Simon, A. (2006) *Working with Children in Care: European Perspectives*, Maidenhead: Open University Press.
Taylor, C. (2006) *Young People in Care and Criminal Behaviour*, London: Jessica Kingsley Publishers.

References

A National Voice (2002) *Amplify: The Report*, Manchester: A National Voice.
Baldwin, N. and Carruthers, L. (1998) *Developing Neighbourhood Support and Child Protection Strategies: The Henley Safe Children Project*, London: Ashgate.
Baldwin, N. and Spencer, N. (1993) Deprivation and child abuse: implications for strategic planning in children's services, *Children & Society*, 7 (4): 357–75.
Big Issue (2001) 10th birthday survey, *Big Issue*, September.
Brewer, M., Muriel, A., Phillips, D. and Sibieta, L. (2009) *Poverty in the UK*, London: Institute for Fiscal Studies.
Child Poverty Action Group (CPAG) (2008) *Child Poverty: The Stats: Analysis of the Latest Poverty Statistics*, London: CPAG.
Cusik, L., Martin, A. and May, T. (2003) *Vulnerability and Involvement in Drug Use and Sex Work*. London: Home Office.
Department of Children, Schools and Families (DCSF) (2008a) *Children looked after in England (including adoption and care leavers) year ending 31 March 2008*. DCSF available at http://www.dcsf.gov.uk/rsgateway/DB/SFR/s000810/index.shtml (accessed 18 September 2009).
—— (2008b) *Outcome Indicators for Children Looked After*, London: DCSF.
—— (2008c) *Permanent and Fixed Exclusions from Schools and Exclusion Appeals in England 2006/07*, London: DCSF.

Department for Health (DH) (2003) *Children Looked After by Local Authorities*, London: DH.

Devaney, J. (2009) Chronic child abuse: the characteristics and careers of children caught in the child protection system, *British Journal of Social Work*, 39 (1): 24–45.

Elliott, L. and Curtis, P. (2009) UK's income gap widest since 60s, *Guardian*, 8 May. Available online at: http://www.guardian.co.uk/society/2009/may/08/poverty-britain-incomes-poor (accessed 8 May 2009).

Ferguson, I. and Lavalette, M. (2009) Social work after 'Baby P', *International Socialism*, 122, Spring: 115–31.

Ford, T., Vostanis, P., Meltzer, H. and Goodman, R. (2007) Psychiatric disorder among British children looked after by local authorities: comparison with children living in private households, *British Journal of Psychiatry*, 190: 319–25.

Gentleman, A. (2009) State failing to protect children in care, MPs say, *Guardian*, 20 April. Available online at: http://www.guardian.co.uk/society/2009/apr/20/state-failing-children. (accessed 1 September 2009).

Hazel, N., Hagell, A., Liddle, M., Archer, D., Grimshaw, R., and King, J. (2002) *Detention and Training: Assessment of the Detention and Training Order and its Impact on the Secure Estate Across England and Wales*, London: Youth Justice Board.

House of Commons Children, Schools and Families Select Committee (2009) *Looked-after Children Third Report Session 2008–09 Volume 1*, London: The Stationery Office.

Hirsch, D. (2007) *Experiences of Poverty and Educational Disadvantage*, York: Joseph Rowntree Foundation.

Kassem, D. (2006) Education of looked-after children: who cares?, in D. Kassem, E. Mufti and J. Robinson (eds) *Education Studies Issues and Critical Perspectives*, Maidenhead: Open University Press.

—— (2009) Learning from Europe: Social pedagogy and looked-after children, in D. Kassem and D. Garratt (eds) *Exploring Key Issues in Education*, London: Continuum.

Magadi, M. and Middleton, S. (2007) *Severe Child Poverty in the UK*, London: Save the Children.

Morris, J. (2000) *Having Someone Who Cares? Barriers to Change in the Public Care of Children*, London: National Children's Bureau.

National Statistics (2003) *The Mental Health of Young People Looked After by Local Authorities*, London: The Stationery Office.

—— (2004) Families: Dependent Children. Available online at http://www.statistics.gov.uk/cci/nugget_print.asp?ID=1163 (accessed 30 April 2009).

Petrie, P., Boddy, J., Cameron, C., Wigfall, C. and Simon, A. (2006) *Working with Children in Care: European Perspectives*, Maidenhead: Open University Press.

Prison Reform Trust (2008) *Bromley Briefings December 2008*. Available online at: http://www.prisonreformtrust.org.uk/subsection.asp?id=1781 (accessed 14 April 2009).

Richardson J. and Lelliott, P. (2003) Mental health needs of looked after children, *Advances in Psychiatric Treatment*, 9 (4): 249–51.

Schmid, M., Golbeck, L., Nuetzel, J. and Fegert, J. (2008) Prevalence of mental disorders among adolescents in German youth welfare institutions, *Child and Adolescent Psychiatry and Mental Health*, 2 (2): 1–8.

The Scottish Government (2008) *Children Looked After Statistics*, Edinburgh: The Scottish Government.

Social Exclusion Unit (SEU) (1999) *Teenage Pregnancy*. London, SEU.

—— (2002) *Reducing Re-offending by Ex-prisoners*. London, SEU.

—— (2003) *A Better Education for Children in Care*. London, SEU.

Statham, J., Candappa, M. Simon, A. and Owen, C. (2002) *Trend in Care: Exploring Reasons for the Increase in Looked After Children by Local Authorities*, London: Thomas Coram Research Unit, Institute of Education, University of London.

Sutton Trust (2006) *The Social Composition of Top Comprehensive School Rates of Eligibility for Free School Meals at the 200 Highest Performing Comprehensive Schools*, London: Sutton Trust.

Taylor, C. (2006) *Young People in Care and Criminal Behaviour*, London: Jessica Kingsley Publishers.

Times Educational Supplement (2005) 23 December 2005.

Verkaik, R. (2009) Children in jail: lottery of justice revealed, *Independent*, 12 May.

Voice for the Child in Care (1998) *Sometimes You've Got to Shout to be Heard*, Introduction, London: Voice for the Child in Care.

Welsh Assembly Government (2008) *Adoptions, Outcomes and Placements for Children Looked After by Local Authorities: Year Ending 31 March 2008*, Cardiff: Welsh Assembly Government.

Wilkinson, R. and Pickett, K. (2009) *The Spirit Level: Why More Equal Societies Almost Always Do Better*, London: Penguin Books.

Wrigley, T. (2009) Academies: the privatization of education, in D. Kassem and D. Garratt (eds) *Exploring Key Issues in Education*, London: Continuum.

3.4 Healthy in body, healthy in mind

John Harrison

And sleep as I in childhood sweetly slept:
Untroubling and untroubled where I lie;
The grass below – above the vaulted sky.
      — From 'I Am' by John Clare

Activity 3.4.1: Mental health issues and you

•   Before reading this chapter write down your feelings and knowledge of mental health issues.

•   Once you have read the chapter review the notes you made. Have your views changed? If so, in what way? If not, can you explain why?

This chapter introduces the issue of children's mental health. It will define mental health and look at how mental health problems manifest in the young. An exploration of the causes and presentations of mental illness will be followed by a discussion of the stigmas faced by those children who have a mental health problem and the chapter will conclude with a critical examination of the treatment services available within the United Kingdom.

Defining mental health

What is mental health? This is a question that raises a number of issues and has led to heated debates among the professionals responsible for the care and treatment of those who suffer with mental health problems. The irrefutable fact is that each of us possesses mental health in the same way that we are either well or ill physically. The crux of the argument rests in what forms this illness, or mental ill health, takes and more importantly for us, how it can manifest in childhood.

John Clare, whose poem opens this chapter, spent most of his adult life being treated for mental illness and lived out his days within what was termed a lunatic asylum under the care of doctors. Yet, elements of the medical profession itself have provided the strongest opponents of the notion of mental illness as a treatable concrete reality. The American psychiatrist Thomas Szasz (1961) theorized that mental illness rather than being a tangible, quantifiable reality is rather the manifestation of human society. According to Szasz, mental illness serves two main functions; first, it allows society to explain those individuals who do not conform to its desired norms and second, it increases the position of the doctor as a figure of responsibility. If the deviant actions of an individual are deemed due to mental illness it provides the society with an explanation that does not require too much introspection. The person is not acting against an unjust society that should be challenged, rather they are mentally ill and that society provides the solution in the form of the doctor in order that the individual can once again think as others do (Foucault 1961). The doctor not only provides the solution in the form of treatment, they are the gatekeepers of what is deemed acceptable in the form of sanity and insanity.

Thus, everybody wins. Society is protected from those who disagree with its core values, the doctor is given a position of authority with all the associated benefits, and last but not least, the 'patient' is able to be legitimately rehabilitated and reintegrated. As a society alters, then what passes for mental illness changes also (Porter 2002). Homosexuality was once seen as a mental illness and would be treated as such by doctors, a concept that the majority of today's society would find hard to accept. In the same way, anorexia nervosa has been recently seen by some as a lifestyle choice even though the majority of doctors would describe it as a mental illness (Chesley, *et al.* 2003).

Indeed, for many in the medical profession mental ill health can be easily identified according to the presentation or symptoms that are particular to an illness. Roth's (1986) response to authors such as Szasz was based around the observation that particular mental health problems have universal symptomologies regardless of the society they present in. Rather, it is the unique nature of each society that dictates how a condition is interpreted (Barry and Green 1992).

Therefore, with this acknowledgement in mind, a definition of what mental health is, for the purpose of this chapter, rather than being society specific should encompass all societies. The definition of mental health and thus mental ill health used here is that used by the World Health Organization, a body dedicated to the treatment of illness in all human communities: 'Mental health is not just the absence of mental disorder. It is a state of well being in which every individual realises his or her own potential' (Herrman, *et al.* 2005).

With this definition and with our earlier acknowledgement that mental health is a universal state experienced by all, we thus need to explore how its absence or alteration can affect the young. Although this chapter is entitled 'Healthy in body, healthy in mind', a possible alternative could have been 'Children's mental ill health'. By exploring the way certain mental illnesses present, we shall be able to measure their impact on the lives of children. The examination of their cause shall provide an understanding of how the modern world can affect the mental health of children (Ciarrochi and Heaven 2008).

Issues specific to childhood

While mental illness can affect any of us at some stage in our lives (Royal College of Psychiatrists 2008b), childhood presents a unique component that needs to be considered before any diagnosis can be made. Before we can identify abnormal mental health in a child, the normal functioning for a child for that age must be established. What is normal behaviour for a child of one age could be the indication of a mental health problem in one older or younger (Barker 1995). Indeed, while some mental health problems such as post-traumatic stress disorder have very specific causes, there is often a developmental issue in a large number of conditions (Swanson and Wadhwa 2008; Harrison 2004). There is not sufficient space within this chapter to explore child development in detail and further reading on the process of development itself would provide a sound understanding of what constitutes normalcy as a child progresses from infancy to adulthood.

Acknowledgement that each of these stages poses particular challenges to the young is needed (Hughes and Graham 2002). Adolescence for instance brings a raft of not only physical changes but an alteration of the young person's status both in and outside the family. Consequentially, conditions such as anorexia nervosa are often diagnosed during adolescence and in some cases are felt to be a response to the challenges of being a teenager.

Another issue to consider is the culture in which the child is developing. While this chapter deals in the main with issues in the United Kingdom, a number of studies have acknowledged the complexities of mental health diagnosis within a multicultural society (Hodes 2000; Appleton and Hammond-Rowley 2000). Awareness and sensitivity are needed when exploring the mental health needs of children from other cultures and a good deal of research remains to be done in this important area.

The causes of mental illness in the young

While the issues of culture and development have already been discussed we need to turn our attention to what may actually cause a mental illness in a child or young person. Before this is undertaken, it is important to firstly acknowledge that mental illness is complex. Many conditions have what are described as multi-factorial causes that require in-depth exploration before any treatment can be undertaken (Zubrick, *et al.* 2001). As a result of this, it is not possible to examine the causes of each mental illness in turn within the confines of this chapter. Instead, the overarching causes of mental illness in the young shall be examined in turn and certain conditions used as illustrations of this.

Genetic and birth factors

Genetic or inherited factors deal with conditions that are specifically developed before the child is born and are often caused by the genetic make-up of the parents. An example of this is the chromosome abnormality called Fragile X, which can result in learning and social impairment and certain physical abnormalities (Turner, *et al.* 1996). Other conditions include foetal alcohol syndrome in which both the physical and mental health of the child are affected by high levels of alcohol consumed by the mother prior to birth (Armstrong 2003).

Physical disease and injury

Physical injury can have a profound impact upon the way mental health develops in the young. Brain injury and illness in particular can greatly affect the cognitive functioning of a child and lead to alterations in behaviour and personality (Fink, *et al.* 2003).

However, it is not just brain injury that can lead to mental health problems. All physical illness can impact upon our mental well-being, and in some cases lead to severe psychiatric illness. If we consider those children who have to spend a protracted period in hospital then issues of social development arise (Royal College of Psychiatrists 2008a). Other conditions may cause alterations in appearance that may lead to loss of self-confidence and depression during a period in life in which great emphasis is placed on appearance (Kahana 2006).

The family

Families play a vital part in the development of the individual. Alongside genetic factors, our childhood upbringing is the main influence in shaping adult identity and personality (Wolff 1989). Although the actual make-up of families differs according to factors such as number of siblings, access to the extended family and the age of parents, it is important that the child is raised in a loving accepting environment with clear boundaries. As the child ages, these boundaries should be altered to accommodate increased cognitive development and a growing understanding of the social world (Barker 1995).

Providing the right 'age appropriate' parenting techniques is a complex process and one that large numbers of parents find difficult. The correct relationship with a younger child may seem stifling and cause developmental delays if applied to a pre-adolescent (Black and Cottrell 1993). These difficulties can be compounded by the parents themselves and a number of studies have identified issues such as poor parental mental health as a significant factor in preventing rounded development (Cleaver, *et al.* 1999). Parents who suffer high degrees of substance addiction often have difficulty in providing secure environments for their children. The nature of both drug and alcohol misuse can result in chaotic home environments in which appropriate adult role models are absent (Gopfert, *et al.* 2004).

As a result, many children lack a stable adult figure with which to build a lasting relationship. Research into the phenomenon has identified clear links between disruptive home environments and conditions such as conduct disorders. What is of particular concern is that a number of children who are raised in chaotic families often lack essential parenting skills themselves and thus have dysfunctional relationships with their own children that require support from outside agencies (Webster-Stratton and Herbert 1994).

The loss of a parent through either divorce or death can also have a lasting, negative impact on a child's mental health. It should also be acknowledged that in a number of cases, separation of the parents may benefit the children. Rather than being exposed to constant fighting between parents the child is able to be brought up in a home environment that is much more stable. Indeed, large numbers of children quickly adjust to reconstituted families with little or no ill effects (Royal College of Psychiatrists 2008c).

However, for some children such separations cause a good deal of mental anguish. The child may blame themselves for the separation or feel that they are no longer loved by either or both parents. Such feelings can quickly develop into low self-esteem and indeed depression as the child attempts to come to terms with the changes in family dynamics. Similar emotions can be experienced by those children who suffer the loss of a parent. Again, guilt for the death of the parent may occur alongside issues of abandonment and fear that the remaining parent may die. In some cases, children develop ritualistic, compulsive behaviours which they believe will keep the rest of the family safe from harm (Velting and Albano 2001). More common are feelings of anxiety when separated from the parent leading to limited social and educational exposure.

Environmental factors

Outside the family, education plays an important part in our development. Not only does schooling equip the child with knowledge, it provides a solid grounding in the social norms and mores of their society (Jenks, *et al.* 1998). The school experience can greatly impact on the social and academic development of the child, with adverse experiences leading to feelings of low self-worth, which in turn manifest themselves in negative and self-destructive patterns of behaviour (Place, *et al.* 2000). Issues such as emotional and behavioural difficulties and school refusal can leave a lasting legacy on how well an individual is integrated into a society, with research identifying a link between difficult behaviour in school and eventual involvement with the criminal justice system (Trupin, *et al.* 2002).

Closely linked to the above is the issue of the environment in which childhood takes place. Research has shown that if a child lives in an area in which there are high levels of drug and alcohol abuse then they a more likely to become involved in such behaviours (Barnard 2007). Poor housing and limited facilities have also been linked to high incidences of depressive illness among young people and to an increase in suicidal behaviours (Agerbo 2003). Less common within this country are factors such as war and natural disasters which have a clear link to mental illness among children. When events such as wars take place, it is often the most vulnerable who suffer first and longest and this normally means children (Everett and Gallop 2001). Such children often develop very particular symptoms, closely linked to their traumatic experiences, which make normal development difficult (Hodes 2000). Within our own society there are other factors that affect the mental health of the young. The media is often cited as being responsible for influencing how children view themselves as well as the world around them. In particular, the media obsession with being thin and a supposed ideal body shape has been felt to be linked to eating disorders such as anorexia nervosa as young women in particular see a link between thinness and acceptance (Peterson, *et al.* 2007). Each of these factors may not be the sole reason for the onset of mental illness in children, but they have been identified as the main reasons behind the young displaying symptoms of mental distress. How this distress manifests itself is explored in the next section.

Symptoms of mental illness

As stated above, this chapter is designed to provide an introduction to children's mental health. Therefore, it is not possible to examine how mental illness can present in great detail; rather each of the main categories or 'classifications' of mental illness will be explored in turn and their main features briefly explained. Before doing so, it is necessary that we understand what classifications are. As indicated, mental health is complex, thus it is vital that a system is established that will allow for ease of identification. Classifications are based around symptoms and causes of a condition. This aids those caring for the child in the diagnosis and treatment of the condition. Rather than dealing with each individual child in turn, the grouping of symptoms allows for a sharing of knowledge among clinicians and provides an indication of prevalence, thus increasing the likelihood of a successful cure (Black and Cottrell 1993).

Disorders of development

The conditions within this classification often deal with the child's ability to communicate with others and interact in age-appropriate ways within given social environments. Speech and other forms of communication can be affected, which often are lacking in emotion and the child may in severe cases have very limited patterns of communication (Hart and Whalon 2008). In tandem with such problems the child may have difficulties in a range of social settings that become more evident as they age and greater expectations are placed upon them. The result may be solitary behaviours, with some children spending time on one particular topic rather than playing with others (Beaumont and Sofronoff 2008). In some instances the child may develop the need for very fixed routines of behaviour such as wearing the same clothes and eating the same food on a daily basis, placing a great strain on families. Although the number of conditions that are encompassed within this classification are extensive, the two most widely known are *autism* and *Asperger's syndrome*.

Emotional disorders

These disorders can be seen to encompass areas such as anxiety, phobias, somatic disorders and obsessive compulsive behaviours. Anxiety is a normal part of human existence. We each experience anxious moments in our lives, before an exam for instance, and this can actually benefit the individual in helping to concentrate on the task ahead. However, when these anxieties prevent normal activities then intervention is needed. The child may complain of physical symptoms such as stomach and headaches without any physical cause. Sleeplessness and other behaviours such as bed-wetting (*enuresis*) may develop and attendance at school may decline as the child is anxious when separated from parents (Lewinsohn, *et al.* 2008).

Phobias are a common condition and many of us can describe a situation or object that will cause us to feel uneasy. Often these feelings have no credence in reality and we may act out of proportion toward the threat posed by the object (King, *et al.* 2005). A problem occurs when the phobia hinders the child's social development. In some cases, this can lead to the avoidance of places where the phobic object can be found, leading to social isolation. Emotional anxieties, as we have seen, may be expressed through physical symptoms such as headaches. In a small number of children this can develop into more complex conditions such as paralysis and loss of vision (Henningson 2005). While there is no physical cause, the child is not consciously choosing to be ill and the treatment of such conditions requires a prolonged and sensitive input from clinicians (Nickel and Egle 2004).

Imagination and imaginative play are an important part of childhood. It is very common for young children to ascribe magical properties to certain actions or objects. However, if these behaviours or rituals increase in frequency and importance then obsessive and intrusive thoughts may develop (Cameron 2007). For instance, a child may believe that they must repeatedly check that a door is closed to prevent injury occurring to a member of the family. Other compulsions include repeated handwashing to prevent the contraction of serious illness (Evans, *et al.* 1999). Thankfully, the majority of these conditions are rare but when they do occur then can often require prolonged input from services. The types of conditions which fall under this classification include: *school refusal*, *anxiety disorders*, *obsessive compulsive disorder*, and *hysteria*.

Affective disorders

Essentially, affective disorders deal with mood. Each of us experiences changes in how well we feel through the course of each day. It is quite normal to feel happy or sad as the occasion dictates. However, when these feelings are continuous they become problematic. Depressed moods are far more common in children than many people realize (Huinzink, *et al.* 2006). Children may become withdrawn, lose interest in activities that they previously enjoyed and develop feelings of low self-worth. They may even begin to blame themselves for problems experienced by other members of the family. The future seems bleak and they may even develop suicidal feelings (Harrison, *et al.* 2007) Such feelings may lead to episodes of self-harming behaviour in which the child may hurt themselves through cutting their arms and legs; others may ingest substances that they know will make them ill (Anderson, *et al.* 2003). In some cases, such behaviours may result in the young person taking their own life (Houston 2001).

In some cases, often among adolescents, there may be feelings of continuous elation. They are often extremely happy and active and may seem to have boundless energy, often having very little if any sleep. The child may move from one topic to another with great rapidity and become frustrated and even aggressive with others (Hsu 1986). There is the potential to engage in risky impulsive behaviour, speech is rapid, with many grandiose statements and in severe cases the individual may hallucinate (see things which are not there), reinforcing inappropriate behaviour (Laroi, *et al.* 2006). The conditions that are included within this category include *depression* and *bipolar disorder*.

Attention disorders

At a time when we are encouraged to promote exercise among the young, it may seem strange that there are some children who simply have too much energy, to the extent that it can be deemed a mental health problem. Indeed, research has tended to suggest that there has been an increase in children being treated with such symptoms (Salmon and Kemp 2002). These conditions tend to be grouped under the term *attention deficit disorder* or *attention deficit hyperactivity disorder* (ADHD). Children find it hard to concentrate on tasks for any great length of time. They are far more active than other children of the same age, seeming to constantly move around and find it hard to keep still (Adams, *et al.* 2008). Parents may describe a very active child who seems to be unable to adapt to accepted social behaviours and may seem unwilling to accept rules that curtail their behaviour. In many cases, it is the onset of formal education that leads to problems as the child has difficulty in dealing with the regimented regime of the classroom (Frankel and Feinberg 2002). Some behaviours may be situational, in that they are more pronounced in say the home or in school but large numbers of children have a condition that is described as pervasive in that it occurs in all circumstances. Consequently, many parents express difficulty in managing the behaviour of their children and often negative family environments are created (Peris and Hinshaw 2003). As a result of their inability to manage effectively within environments such as education, many children will find themselves labelled as deviant and thus end up with a dual diagnosis with the category given below.

Conduct disorders

Attention disorders are one of the main causes of conduct disorder although a number of others have been identified. In a large number of cases parenting issues have been observed. Home life may be described as chaotic, often with aggressive relationships between family members. Parents may have problems dealing with their child; inconsistent parenting techniques are common, with boundaries of acceptable behaviour often changing (Modesto-Lowe, *et al.* 2008). Supervision of the child may be limited and children are often left to their own devices. As a consequence, the child may become involved in anti-social behaviours that lead in some cases to criminal convictions. Within the category, there are three main conditions: *oppositional defiant disorder, socialized conduct disorder* and *unsocialized conduct disorder*. In essence these all deal with the same range of behaviours but there are some important differences. First, oppositional defiant disorder is often found in younger children. While behaviours may include refusing to follow the requests of adults and disruption, they are often less severe in nature (Mireault, *et al.* 2008). Socialized conduct disorder is often characterized by aggressive, anti-social acts such as bullying and stealing. However, the child is often in a close relationship with a peer group who behave in the same way. Authority figures such as parents and teachers are often confronted and there is a strong link between this condition and criminal behaviours (Fergusson and Horwood 1998). Unsocialized conduct disorder is similar in terms of the actions of the child but the difference lies in their inability to form relationships with other children. Often the child has difficulty in social situations and spends a good deal of time alone or with younger children (Vostanis, *et al.* 2003). In some very serious cases, the child may engage in behaviours such as fire-starting and cruelty to animals.

The outcome for a number of children with such a diagnosis is often poor, with serious mental health problems occurring in adulthood.

Other clinical conditions

We have concentrated on the main categories of mental illness affecting the young. As indicated, there is not enough space within this chapter to explore many others in the detail they deserve. Conditions such as the eating disorders *anorexia nervosa* and *bulimia nervosa* are often seen in the young. Others such as *enuresis* and *encopresis* (faecal soiling) are often exclusive to children. Children may in a small number of cases also be susceptible to illness more common in adults such as *schizophrenia* and further reading is recommended to explore these issues in the detail they require. Yet, whatever diagnosis a child receives they must deal with the treatment of the condition and the acknowledgement that within our society, mental illness continues to be stigmatized.

A question of stigma

Attitudes towards mental illness have always been part of any society. In some ways how a culture dealt with mental illness was an indication of the society itself. In the past people with mental health problems have been seen as being possessed by demons or endowed with special gifts of prophecy and have been treated accordingly (Porter 2002).

Activity 3.4.2: Attitudes to mental illness

After reading this chapter ask friends, family and colleagues what they feel about mental health issues.

- What do they understand by mental health disorders?
- What chance is there, do they think, that they will ever suffer from a mental health problem (research the statistics)?
- Would they ever have a relationship with someone who had had a mental health problem?

Ask each person to justify their answers. Can you explain their responses?

We would expect our modern society to have a greater understanding of those with mental health problems. However, it may come as a shock to learn that the Royal College of Psychiatrists launched the 'Changing Minds' campaign to reduce the stigmas associated with mental ill health. This coincided with a range of other initiatives in the acknowledgement that many of those who suffer a mental illness are at the margins of our communities. What appears evident is the fact that the majority of people have little understanding of what mental illness is and how it can affect people. As a consequence, the mentally ill are often labelled as 'crazy' or 'loony' and made to feel that they have less right to human dignity than the rest of the population. Such perceptions seem to resonate throughout all aspects of our society, with one study showing that even children's cartoons show the mentally ill in a way described as 'disrespectful' (Hinshaw 2006).

While more work is needed in this area, it is of interest to note that the Royal College of Psychiatrists campaign does not actually deal with mental illnesses common in children, despite the fact that research has shown that children with mental health problems are viewed negatively by the rest of the population (Pescosolido, *et al.* 2007). Indeed, the problem of mental health stigma among the young is so great that some have difficulty accessing the treatments they need (Funderburk, *et al.* 2007).

Activity 3.4.3: Mental health services for young people

- Explore the level of mental health services available to young people in your area.
- What is available and does it meet the needs of your local community?
- It might be useful to start at your local GP's surgery. What mental health services are provided there? How accessible are they? Is there provision specifically aimed at young people?

Treatment issues

The treatment of children and adolescents with mental health problems has become an important political issue in recent years. In September 2004, the Children's National Service Framework placed improved child mental health as one of its 11 standards for improving the lives of children. A systematic review of treatment services was undertaken in November 2008 as part of the government's Children's Plan. The mental well-being of the young within the United Kingdom would seem to have been secured. Yet, a number of problems have been identified and away from official policy deficiencies appear to exist. Before these are discussed, a brief overview of treatment services will be given. As with causes and symptoms, there is not the room to offer more than a framework of what is available. Although there is no uniform system across the entire country, Child and Adolescent Mental Health Services (CAMHS) can be divided into four main sections or tiers.

- *Tier One*: These are services offered by those who are not mental health professionals. While they may offer basic treatments for minor problems as well as health promotion and general advice, they are often the referral agencies for more in-depth treatment. They include general practitioners, school nurses, social workers and teachers.
- *Tier Two*: Working mainly in the primary care sector, these are specialists who often have a formal mental health qualification and include professionals such as counsellors and psychologists.

- *Tier Three*: Dedicated community mental health teams make up the bulk of services in this tier. Mostly based around out-patient treatments, they offer more specialized treatments that may involve long term and multi-agency treatment programmes. Often involved in more complex and severe conditions, staff may include child psychiatrists and specialist children's mental health nurses.
- *Tier Four*: This tier deals with the most severe and challenging conditions. These include specialized day and in-patient centres, eating disorder units and secure forensic adolescent units for those deemed a risk to themselves and others. Again, they are staffed by a range of specially qualified professionals such as psychiatrists and nurses but they may also include play and art therapists, teachers and physiotherapists.

It is important to note that the tiers are not mutually exclusive and a child may be involved in more than one tier at a time.

Such a structured service would suggest that the mental health needs of young people are well catered for in this country. However, an introduction to children's mental health would not be complete without the acknowledgement that problems do exist. It should be accepted that the National Health Service which provides the majority of treatments is not an infinite resource and problems of provision do arise. In recent times, research has highlighted the length of time that children and their families often have to wait for specialized treatment. As a consequence, there is a high rate of patient non-attendance in CAMHS (Terry 2003).

The complex nature of the tier system has also been identified as problematic. A lack of integration between the various tiers and the agencies involved has led to a reduction in efficiency (Worrall-Davies and Marino-Francis 2008). Other problems include a lack of specialized education for those in Tier One. School nurses, who are often the first to be alerted to mental health issues in children, have complained of a lack of training (Leighton, *et al.* 2003). Research has also identified concerns among ethnic minorities, who feel a blanket approach to treatment fails to acknowledge cultural differences (Clarke 2003).

While the recent independent review has made a number of suggestions to improve treatment conditions, only time will tell if these concerns are dealt with. In the meantime, large numbers of children continue to be referred for treatment (Royal College of Psychiatrists 2008c).

Conclusion

This chapter intended to provide an introduction to a very complex topic. It is complex because we ourselves are complex and mental health is about each of us. As we have seen, the concept of mental illness itself is not as transparent as first assumed and each culture's attitude toward the phenomenon should be taken into consideration. While we have looked at the main conditions and causes of mental illness in children, further exploration is recommended and the websites given below provide a suitable staging post.

http://www.youngminds.com
http://www.rcpsych.ac.uk

Student reflection

Having read this chapter, consider the treatment of child mental illness in the UK.

- What more do you think can be done to help children who suffer for mental ill health?

Key points

- Each of us possesses mental health and what is termed mental illness is complex and has changed over time.
- Mental health can be defined as mental well-being and the fulfilment of potential.
- In order to identify mental ill health in the young, normalcy, in terms of stages of development, must be established.
- There are many causes of mental illness in the young. These include genetic and birth factors, physical disease or injury, the family and environmental factors (school, housing, the media, war etc.)
- There are many classifications of disorders which affect the mental health of the young. These include disorders of development, emotional disorders, affective disorders, attention disorders and conduct disorders.
- There are a number of stigmas attached to mental illness. These can include negative language and difficulty in accessing the necessary treatment due to the stigma involved.
- Current treatment for children's mental health is via Children and Adolescent Mental Health Services (CAMHS). CAMHS operates through four tiers however this has led to issues such as the level of specialized training for those professionals working at Tier One.
- Further issues surrounding CAMHS include the length of time children must wait for treatment and patient non-attendance.

Recommended reading

Barker, P. (2004) *Basic Child Psychiatry*, 7th edn, London: Blackwell.
Dwivedi, K. and Harper, P. (2004) *Promoting Emotional Well Being of Children and Adolescents and Preventing Their Mental Ill Health*, London: Jessica Kingsley.
Goodman, R. and Scott, S. (2005) *Child Psychiatry*, London: Blackwell.
Royal College of Psychiatrists (2008) *Reading Lights*, London: Royal College of Psychiatrists.

References

Adams, Z., Derefinko, K., Milich, R. and Fillmore, M. (2008) Inhibitory functioning across ADHD subtypes: recent findings, clinical implications and future directions, *Developmental Disabilities Research Review*, 14: 268–75.
Agerbo, E. (2003) Unemployment and suicide, *Journal of Epidemiology and Community Health*, 57: 560–1.
Anderson, M., Standen, P. and Noon, J. (2003) Nurses and doctors perceptions of young people who engage in suicidal behaviour: a contemporary grounded theory analysis, *International Journal of Nursing Studies*, 40: 587–97.
Appleton, P. and Hammond-Rowley, S. (2000) Addressing the population burden of child and

adolescent mental health problems: a primary care model, *Child Psychology and Psychiatry Review*, 5: 9–16.

Armstrong, E. (2003) *Conceiving Risk, Bearing Responsibility: Foetal Alcohol Syndrome and the Diagnosis of Moral Disorder*, New York: Johns Hopkins University Press.

Barker, P. (1995) *Basic Child Psychiatry*, London: Blackwell.

Barnard, M. (2007) *Drug Addiction and Families*, London: Jessica Kingsley.

Barry, M. and Greene, S. (1992) Implicit models of mental disorder: a qualitative approach to the delineation of public attitudes, *Irish Journal of Psychology*, 13: 141–60.

Beaumont, R. and Sofronoff, K. (2008) A multi-component social skills intervention for children with Asperger's syndrome: the Junior Detective Training Programme, *Journal of Child Psychology and Psychiatry*, 49: 743–53.

Black, D. and Cottrell, D. (1993) *Seminars in Child and Adolescent Psychiatry*, London: Gaskill.

Cameron, C. (2007) Obsessive-compulsive disorder in children and adolescents, *Journal of Psychiatric and Mental Health Nursing*, 14: 196.

Chesley, E., Alberts, J., Klien, J. and Kreipe, R. (2003) Pro or con? Anorexia nervosa and the Internet, *Journal of Adolescent Health*, 32: 123–4.

Ciarrochi, J. and Heaven, P. (2008) Learned social hopelessness: the role of explanatory style in predicting social support during adolescence, *Journal of Child Psychology and Psychiatry*, 49: 1279–86.

Clarke, J. (2003) Developing separate mental health services for minority ethnic groups: what changes are needed? *Mental Health Practice*, 6: 22–6.

Cleaver, H., Unell, I. and Aldgate, J. (1999) *Children's Needs – Parenting Capacity: The Impact of Parental Mental Illness, Alcohol, Drug Use and Domestic Violence on Children's Development*, London: The Stationery Office.

Department for Children, Schools and Families (2008) *The Children's Plan: Building Brighter Futures*, London: The Stationery Office.

Department of Health (2004) *National Service Framework for Children, Young People and Maternity Services: The Mental Health and Psychological Well Being of Children and Young People*, London: The Stationery Office.

Evans, D., Gray, L. and Leckman, J. (1999) The rituals, fears and phobias of young children: insights from developmental psychopathology and neurobiology, *Child Psychiatry and Human Development*, 29: 261–76.

Everett, B. and Gallop, R. (2001) *The Link between Childhood Trauma and Mental Illness*, London: Sage.

Fergusson, D. and Horwood, J. (1998) Early conduct problems and later life opportunities, *Journal of Child Psychology and Psychiatry*, 39: 1097–1109.

Fink, P., Hansen, M., Sondergaard, L. and Fydenberg, M. (2003) Mental illness in new neurological patients, *Journal of Neurology, Neurosurgery and Psychiatry*, 74: 819.

Foucault, M. (1961) *Madness and Civilization*, London: Routledge.

Frankel, F. and Feinberg, D. (2002) Social problems associated with ADHD vs. ODD in children referred for friendship problems, *Child Psychiatry and Human Development*, 33: 125–46.

Funderburk, J., McCormick, B. and Austin, J. (2007) Does attitude toward epilepsy mediate the relationship between perceived stigma and mental health outcomes in children with epilepsy?, *Epilepsy and Behaviour*, 11: 71–6.

Gopfert, M., Webster, P. and Seeman, M. (2004) *Parental Psychiatric Disorder: Distressed Parents and their Families*, Cambridge: Cambridge University Press.

Harrison, J. (2004) Mental health, in D. Wyze (ed.) *Childhood Studies: An Introduction*, London: Blackwell.

Harrison, J., Crosby, C. and Jonker, C. (2007) The development and piloting of an instrument to measure care staff attitudes toward child self-harm, *Vulnerable Children and Youth Studies*, 2: 232–45.

Hart, J. and Whalon, K. (2008) Promote academic engagement and communication of students with autism spectrum disorder in inclusive settings, *Interaction in School and Clinic*, 44: 116–20.

Henningsen, P. (2005) Medically unexplained physical symptoms, anxiety and depression: a meta-analytic review, *Psychosomatic Medicine*, 67: 111–15.

Herrman, H., Saxena, S., Moodie, R. and Walker, L. (2005) Promoting mental health as a public health priority. In *Promoting Mental Health: concepts, emerging evidence, practice*, Geneva: World Health Organization.

Hinshaw, P. (2006) *The Mark of Shame: Stigma of Mental Illness*, Oxford: Oxford University Press.

Hodes, M. (2000) Psychologically distressed refugee children in the United Kingdom, *Child Psychology and Psychiatry Review*, 5: 57–68.

Houston, K. (2001) Suicide in young people aged 15–24: a psychological autopsy study, *Journal of Affective Disorders*, 63: 159–70.

Hughes, C. and Graham, A. (2002) Measuring executive functions in childhood: problems and solutions?, *Child and Adolescent Mental Health*, 7: 131–43.

Huinzink, A., Ferdinand, R., van der Ende, J. and Verhulst, F. (2006) Symptoms of anxiety and depression in children and use of MDMA, *British Medical Journal*, 332: 825–7.

Hsu, L. (1986) Mania in adolescence, *Journal of Clinical Psychiatry*, 47: 596–9.

Jenks, C., James, A. and Prout, A. (1998) *Theorising Childhood*, Cambridge: Polity Press.

Kahana, S. (2006) Posttraumatic stress in youth experiencing illness and injuries, *Traumatology*, 12: 148–61.

King, N., Muris, P. and Ollendick, T. (2005) Childhood fears and phobias: assessment and treatment, *Child and Adolescent Mental Health*, 10: 50–6.

Laroi, F., Van der Linden, M. and Goeb, J. (2006) Hallucinations and delusions in children and adolescents, *Current Psychiatry Review*, 4: 473–85.

Leighton, S., Worraker, A. and Nolan, P. (2003) School nurses and mental health, *Mental Health Practice*, 7: 14–20.

Lewinsohn, P., Holm-Demona, J., Small, J., Seely, J. and Joiner, T. (2008) Separation anxiety disorder in childhood as a risk factor for future mental illness, *Journal of American Academic Child and Adolescent Psychiatry*, 47: 548–55.

Mireault, G., Rooney, S., Kouwenhoven, K. and Hannan, C. (2008) Oppositional behaviour and anxiety in boys and girls: a cross sectional study in two community samples, *Child Psychiatry and Human Development*, 39: 519–27.

Modesto-Lowe, V., Danforth, J. and Brooks, D. (2008) ADHD: does parenting style matter? *Clinical Paediatrics*, 47: 865–72.

Nickel, R. and Egle, U. (2004) Psychosomatic therapy in somatization disorders, *Journal of Psychosomatic Research*, 56: 591–5.

Pescosolido, B., Perry, B., Martin, J., McLeod, J. and Jenson, P. (2007) Stigmatizing attitudes and beliefs about treatment and psychiatric medications for children with mental illness, *Psychiatric Services*, 58: 613–18.

Peris, T. and Hinshaw, S. (2003) Family dynamics and pre-adolescent girls with ADHD: the relationship between expressed emotion, ADHD symptomotology and co-morbid disruptive behaviour, *Journal of Child Psychology and Psychiatry*, 44: 1177–91.

Place, M., Wilson, J., Martin, E. and Hulsmeir, J. (2000) The frequency of emotional and behavioural disturbance in an EBD school, *Child Psychology and Psychiatry Review*, 5: 76–80.

Porter, R. (2002) *Madness: A Brief History*, Oxford: Oxford University Press.

Roth, M. and Kroll, J. (1986) *Reality of Mental Illness*, Cambridge: Cambridge University Press.

Royal College of Psychiatrists (2008a) *Surviving Adolescence*, London: Royal College of Psychiatrists.

—— (2008b) *When Bad Things Happen*, London: Royal College of Psychiatrists.

—— (2008c) *Child and Adolescent Psychiatrists: How They Can Help*, London: Royal College of Psychiatrists.

Salmon, G. and Kemp, A. (2002) ADHD: a survey of psychiatric and paediatric practice, *Child and Adolescent Mental Health*, 7: 73–8.

Swanson, J. and Wadhwa, P. (2008) Developmental origins of child mental health disorders, *Journal of Child Psychology and Psychiatry*, 49: 1009–19.

Szasz, T. (1961) *The Myth of Mental Illness*, London: Secker and Warbury.

Terry, J. (2003) Brief intervention: a pilot in initiative in a child and adolescent mental health service, *Mental Health Practice*, 6: 18–20.

Trupin, E., Stewart, D., Beach, B. and Boesky, L. (2002) Effectiveness of a dialectical behaviour therapy program for incarcerated female juvenile offenders, *Child and Adolescent Mental Health*, 7: 121–8.

Turner, G., Webb, T., Wake, S. and Robinson, H. (1996) The prevalence of fragile X syndrome, *American Journal of Medical Genetics*, 64: 196–7.

Velting, O. and Albano, A. (2001) Current trends in the understanding and treatment of social phobia in youth, *Journal of Child Psychology and Psychiatry*, 42: 127–40.

Vostanis, P., Meltzer, H., Goodman, R. and Ford, T. (2003) Service utilization by children with conduct disorders, *European Child and Adolescent Psychiatry*, 5: 231–8.

Webster-Stratton, C. and Herbert, M. (1994) *Troubled Families, Problem Children*, London: Wiley-Blackwell.

Wolff, S. (1989) *Childhood and Human Nature: The Development of Personality*. Routledge: London.

Worrall-Davies, A. and Marino-Francis, F. (2008) Eliciting children's and young people's views of child and adolescent mental health services: a systematic review of best practice, *Child and Adolescent Mental Health*, 13: 9–15.

World Health Organization website: http://www.who.int/en/

Zubrick, S., Silburn, S. and Williams, A. (2001) Promotion and prevention in mental health, *Healthway News*, May: 6–8.

Part 4

The politics of childhood

> Children today are tyrants. They contradict their parents, gobble their food, and tyrannize their teachers.
>
> — Socrates

The above quote attributed to Socrates (469–399 BC) suggests that concern around the declining moral standards of youth is not a new phenomenon. However, recent media 'scaremongering', supported by government rhetoric, particularly through the 'respect' agenda, has ensured that teenage behaviour is an issue of major public debate.

Robinson's chapter examines the construction of the modern folk devil – the hoodie, suggesting that the hoodie is, in fact, a reinvention of a familiar, traditionally demonized sector of society – the white, working-class and potentially violent youth (Cohen 2002). Robinson highlights that fact that the hoodie, largely a construction of negative and often fervent media discourses, has become a source of societal moral panic.

Using a case study illustration, Robinson suggests that a child may be led to construct their own identity as a member of a counter-culture group, as a hoodie, through school experiences such as low teacher expectations and poor interactions with teachers. Such experiences can engender disengagement with the education system and can, eventually, result in anti-social behaviour. Robinson concludes that the social discourses which create the hoodie are a manifestation of a long-standing age-related discourse by which adults construct the young as incomplete, as adults-in-process. This is what Woodhead (2003) termed a 'developmentalism' approach to children and young people (see Chapter 1.2, this volume). He states that in order to end demonization of the youth we need to reassess the discourse we use to construct them.

Wrigley's chapter explores the high-stakes testing environment of modern schooling and education – one of the factors which may, indeed, cause some children to disengage with the education process due to the labels which testing, or more accurately, failure in testing, can produce for young people. He points out how these labels, which may be assigned in primary education, can impact psychologically to the detriment of young people and affect their futures such as access to secondary or higher education.

Wrigley, citing Foucault (2002), points out the links between assessment and socially validated knowledge and, therefore, between testing and power. After tracing the history of testing from the Victorian period to contemporary society, Wrigley highlights the links between the micromanagement of education via assessment and the marketization of education globally through neoliberal politics and suggests that, in effect, today's high-stakes testing educational environment is a return to 'payment by result' of the 1870 Forster Act.

To conclude, Wrigley suggests that there are alternatives to the high-stakes testing regime in the form of assessment for learning and 'rich tasks'.

Montgomery's chapter, like many others in this volume, deals with a fundamental, though highly controversial area of childhood studies – the rights of the child. Having outlined the approach of the United Nations Convention on the Rights of the Child (UNCRC), including the precept that the child has the same participatory rights in society as the adult, Montgomery notes how many governments do not fulfil this obligation and suggests that the UNCRC may, in fact, present an idealized vision rather than a practical reality. Montgomery uses the effective, though somewhat extreme, example of the rights, or lack thereof, of a premature child to illustrate the tensions between the rights of the child to be listened to as well as to be cared for. Once again we see within this discussion the essential tensions which lie at the heart of most issues relating to childhood dealt within in this volume, such as sexuality, rights, notions of risk and so on. This tension creates what Cunningham (1995: 190) terms contemporary 'confusion' and 'angst' about childhood and it is located in the dichotomy within the adult-world's construction of the child. This dichotomy revolves around public discourses which include both the remnants of the Romantic view of as a child, that is, as in progress of becoming and so, therefore, as dependent, in need and innocent, and discourses which argue that children are persons with their own rights and with a degree of autonomy.

The final chapter in this part deals with a topic which has been high on New Labour's agenda in the UK since their election in 1997 – childhood poverty. Outlining the fact that there is much debate about what constitutes poverty today in Britain, Grant suggests that this debate influences, and may in fact impede, the ways in which poverty is being addressed. Grant states that childhood poverty is different today than it was in the past as today children are not allowed to work to alleviate poverty and to this extent they have even less agency in, or control over, their socio-economic status than they did in previous centuries.

Grant discusses the consequences of childhood poverty such as low educational achievement (see Chapter 2.2, this volume), poor employment prospects and research evidence which illustrates how poverty is pervasive across lifespans. While it is acknowledged that the current government have put into practice measures to attempt to counter-act poverty such as the minimum wage, housing support, focus on parenting skills, the effectiveness across generational cycles of such measures is questioned. It is suggested that radical changes to the policies and instruments being utilized to break the poverty cycle are required if they are going to be successful.

References

Cohen, S. (2002) *Folk Devils and Moral Panics: The Creation of the Mods and Rockers*, 3rd edn, London: Routledge.

Cunningham, H. (1995) *Children and Childhood in Western Society since 1500*, London: Longman.

Foucault, M. (2002) *Essential works of Foucault 1954–84 vol. 3*, J. Faubion (ed.), London: Penguin.

Woodhead, M. (2003) The child in development, in M. Woodhead and H. Montgomery (eds) *Understanding Childhood: An Interdisciplinary Approach*, Chichester: John Wiley/OU.

4.1   The social construction of deviant identities

The devil wears a hoodie

John Robinson

> ['Hoodie' has] made [its] official entrance into the English language, after being included in the 9th edition of the *Collins English Dictionary* [2007]. [It is defined as] 'a young person who wears a hooded sweatshirt, regarded by some as a potential hooligan'.
>
> (Newman 2007)

It does not take more than a cursory glance at the broadcast and print media to recognize that certain social groups are being demonized and presented as outsiders in society. At the time of writing several social groups compete for this 'prize' – adherents of the Islamic faith, East European migrants, travellers and young white males. However, this social *otherizing* is not a new phenomenon.

Activity 4.1.1: The other and otherizing

- What do you think is meant by *otherizing*?
- Research the concept of the other – you might want to start by looking at Jacques Lacan [1964] (1977) *The Four Fundamental Concepts of Psycho-analysis*, London: Hogarth Press.

Byron (2009) reports how a 6,000-year-old Egyptian tomb was inscribed with the following words – 'We live in a decaying age. Young people no longer respect their parents. They are rude and impatient. They frequently inhabit taverns and have no self-control'. This writing and construction of young people through social discourse is re-inscribed throughout history. Bartlett (2008), for example, has reported that hooded tops were also the garment of choice for twelfth-century juvenile delinquents. The teenage apprentice boys of London were lawless, violent and the scourge of the capital. 'They were away from home for seven years with no parental control and they would riot regularly for political and religious reasons' (Bartlett 2008, cited in Clout 2008). Hooded tops were worn by most citizens during medieval winters, according to Bartlett, and they also served to hide the identity of young miscreants. Bawdon (2009) quotes the *Morning Chronicle*, 22 October 1842: 'It is a strange anomaly, that in a country boasting to be the most civilized in the world, no effective machinery exists for checking the growth of vice in young offenders. Our gaols, as reformatories, are worse than useless.' The consequences of the social work that such labelleing does is to create an image of young, particularly white and working-class, males in contemporary society as lawless and feral, to be feared and avoided. Byron (2009) suggests that this process leads to the development of the condition of ephebiphobia – the fear of young people. This is not just a fear felt by adults. Children under ten report how they fear teenagers in public social spaces because of their size and boisterousrness (Engaging Communities Foundation 2006; Bawdon 2009).

This chapter will explore how these social images are presented through the mass media and how these presentations amount to what S. Cohen (1972) referred to as the creation of moral panics through the demonization of folk devils. An account will then be given of how these 'devilish' identities can be amplified through social interactions by analysing the case of one young learner in school. The chapter will conclude by trying to present a contrary argument to this presentation of the 'devils in hoodies'.

Boys will be boys?

The portrayal of teenage boys in the mass media tends to be overwhelmingly negative. Bawdon (2009) conducted research into the presentation of teenagers in the media and into teenagers' responses to how they are constructed in the media. He reports that more than half of the stories about teenage boys in national and regional newspapers in 2008 – that is, 4,374 out of 8,629 – were about crime. The word most commonly used to describe them was 'yobs' (591 times), followed by 'thugs' (254 times), 'sick' (119 times) and 'feral' (96 times). Other terms often used included 'hoodie', 'louts', 'heartless', 'evil', 'frightening', 'scum', 'monsters', 'inhuman' and 'threatening'. Such language used repeatedly builds up a strong social discourse according to which the male youths in our society are defined and constructed.

Bawdon (2009) explains that this negative discourse used to define teenage boys has become so overwhelming that even in areas where we might expect more positive media coverage related to male youth – sport and entertainment – a critical line was usually taken. 'Only 16 per cent of stories about teens and entertainment were positive: only 24 per cent about teens and sport were positive' (Bawdon 2009, cited in Garner 2009).

Shockingly, Bawdon suggested that the best chance a teenager had of receiving sympathetic coverage was if they had died. 'We found some news coverage where teen boys were described in glowing terms – "model student", "angel", "altar boy" or "every mother's perfect son" … but sadly these were reserved for teenage boys who met a violent and untimely death' (Bawdon 2009, cited in Garner 2009).

Bawdon's (2009) report includes details of a survey of nearly 1,000 teenage boys conducted by Echo Research (http://www.echoresearch.com/en/) who found that 85 per cent of those surveyed believed that newspapers portrayed them in a bad light. They felt that reality television – with shows like *The X Factor* and *Britain's Got Talent* – portrayed them in a better light with fewer than 20 per cent believing they were being portrayed negatively. As a result of the negative press, 80 per cent felt adults were more wary of teenage boys now than they had been a year ago. However, the most striking finding, according to Bawdon (2009), was that many were now more wary of boys of their own age. The most popular reason cited for this was media stories, followed by their own or their friends' bad experiences of other teenage boys. 'It seems the endless diet of media reports about "yobs" and "feral" youths is making them fearful of other teens …. Nearly a third said they are "always" or "often" wary of teenage boys they don't know' (Bawdon 2009, cited in Garner 2009).

Garner (2009) notes that nearly three-quarters of those surveyed said that they had changed their behaviour as a result of this wariness. The most common change, cited by 45.7 per cent of those surveyed, was boys avoiding places where teenagers hung around. Others included dressing differently (14.2 per cent), and changing who they were seen with (11.9 per cent).As Bawdon, presenting her research at the British Library in March 2009, put it, 'For much of the press, there is no such thing as a good news story about teenagers …. Media coverage of boys is unrelentingly negative, focusing almost entirely on them as victims or perpetrators of crime' (Garner 2009).

Psychologist and TV presenter Byron (2009) in an article for the *Education Guardian* reported some comments from teenagers concerning the way they feel the public react to them in response to media representations of youth. Below are some of the comments:

'I've had people cross the road to avoid me. It's worse when you're wearing a hoodie. The problem is that people have read all this bad stuff in newspapers. They focus on the small minority of teenagers who get up to things, and the rest of us are tarred with that brush. It's unfair to label us all like that' (Joe White, 16 from Shropshire).

'When you get on public transport, especially if you're in a group, it's like "Uh-oh! They're going to cause trouble!" But we're just like them; we're using the bus or the train because we want to get somewhere' (Anna Godinho, 16 from West London).

'I got on a train with a friend whose dad had bought us first-class tickets. Straight away the guard arrived and was quite rude to us. He just assumed that we were some-where we shouldn't be. He treated us with a total lack of respect' (Charlie d'Auria, 18 from South London).

(quoted in Byron 2009: 2)

Hooded devils …

Stanley Cohen published a seminal study of 'folk devils' and moral panics in 1972, which was subsequently re-issued with a new introduction focusing on the symbols of trouble in 1987 and on moral panics as cultural politics in 2002. This study drew heavily on the sociology of labelling theory within the symbolic interactionist sociology of deviance developed by the Chicago School. One of the main exponents of labelling was Howard Becker (1963):

Social groups create deviance by making the rules whose infraction constitutes devi-ance, and by applying those rules to particular people and labelling them as outsiders. From this point of view, deviance is not a quality of the act the person commits, but rather a consequence of the application by others of the rules and sanctions to an 'offender'. The deviant is the one to whom the label has been successfully applied; deviant behaviour is behaviour that people so label.

(8–9)

What this quotation from Becker reveals is that, first, deviance is a social construct and, second, that as such it illustrates a power relationship in the sense that in order for a label to stick those applying the label must have the power, formal or informal, to make that label stick. Thus the identification of a particular social group as a group of folk devils implies a hierarchical relationship, often based on age, but equally so based on alternative formulations of *otherizing*. The opposition which is perceived as divergent from the norm within a set of binary oppositions is frequently constructed as the other, for example, Christianity/Islam, West/East, homeowner/traveller and, as the other, may be demonized. We will return to the issues that arise out of this differentiation based on age in the conclusion to this chapter.

Cohen (1987) identified three broad strands in the sociological studies of what Albert K. Cohen (1955) referred to as 'the delinquent boys': structural, historical or problems-related studies; cultural, style or solution-related studies; and biographical or lived-experience studies. The first group of studies generally identified a group of youngsters who were fighting back against a system that was not working for them and is exemplified by S. Cohen's (1972) study of working-class culture and Willis's 'lads' in *Learning to Labour* (1978). Here the marginalized groups are described as developing a counter-culture with which to retaliate against the mainstream culture from which they feel excluded.

The second group of studies focused on the symbolic or magical nature of this resistance through the rituals of subculture, drawing on Hall and Jefferson's (1976) *Resistance through Ritual* and Hebdige's (1979) study of the style of British subcultures. The third group of studies focused on biographical locations – school, neighbourhood or work – as the locus for the analysis of 'delinquent' behaviour, such as Corrigan's (1979) study of kids growing up on the street corners of Sunderland.

What these groups of studies show, most notably Willis's (1978) study, is that the lived experiences of those labelled as outsiders (of whatever hue) cannot be understood without locating those lived experiences within the context of an understanding of both structure and agency (Giddens 1979) and that attempts to do so are always going to remain partial. Moreover, the studies highlight the fact that significant social groups appear to be absent from this analysis of recent history, namely over 25s, girls and minority ethnic people. S. Cohen (1972) identifies several elements that are necessary for the processes of demonization of any particular social group: exaggeration and distortion; prediction; symbolization; manufacturing the news; and reaction.

A clear example of these processes of demonization were presented by Channel 4's programme *The Insider* (2009). Rod Morgan, a former advisor to the British government on youth crime, argues that these processes are amplified by the system of police targets established by the Home Office, which are completely unrelated to the seriousness of the offence, so it is easier for officers to meet targets by tackling low-level crime. One police constable seemed to confirm Morgan's concerns. He told *The Insider* that officers are now keen to deal with young people who commit minor crimes in a formal way in order to help them reach their targets. The targets are linked to annual bonuses, so these financial incentives seem to be encouraging officers to give the young people a criminal record rather than dealing with them informally, by giving them a talking-to in front of their parents, for example. This point was re-iterated in a BBC Radio 4 *You and Yours* programme (17 March 2009) which quoted a female police constable's blog.

The police constable on *The Insider* claimed that some officers could be tackling minor crimes instead of investigating more serious offences in order to reach their targets. He told the programme that in some deprived areas, despite the police having intelligence about people involved with potential firearms offences, officers do not take any action because it would require a serious investment of police resources and would not generate as many results to help them reach their targets.In the last four years the number of sentences passed in English and Welsh youth courts has increased by around a quarter. John Fassenfelt, Chief Representative of more than 8,000 youth court magistrates, told

The Insider that he has seen young people in court for stealing a small chocolate bar or fighting in the playground. Once a child has been convicted of an offence in court, he or she automatically goes to court for every subsequent offence they are charged with, no matter how trivial. If they are sentenced on three occasions and then arrested again within three years, they will be automatically categorized as a Persistent Young Offender. Several youths claimed on the programme that they had been stopped three or four times a day since being labelled as Persistent Young Offenders and arrested for crimes they had not committed, just because of their label. A boy of just 11 claimed that he was locked up for three days in a cell on his own. These young people say that this encourages them to carry on committing offences as they are being regarded as criminals. Morgan argues that this kind of police targeting is tantamount to child abuse (*The Insider* 2009). It is these demonizing processes that make the following newspaper comments understandable:

> Enforced conscription is the answer to sick yobs.
> (Sue Carroll in the *Daily Mirror*, 2 March 2009)

> What word other than 'feral' better describes the swarms of hooligans abandoned to their own devices by slattern mothers and absentee 'babyfathers'? No one crosses the road if they spot a crocodile of Boy Scouts coming in the other direction. But nor does anyone in their right mind risk walking through a scrum of hoodies hogging the pavement – not unless they fancy a knife in their ribs .
> (Richard Littlejohn in the *Daily Mail*, 18 November 2008)

> We demonise all boys as feral …. Then wonder why they turn into hoodies.
> (Suzanne Moore in the *Mail on Sunday*, 15 March 2009)

… And moral panics

Cohen (2002: viii) discusses the elusive and somewhat contradictory nature of moral panics created by demonizing sectors of society. He claims that though inconsistent in nature, moral panics are rather predictable. In fact, it may be the very contradictory nature of moral panics that makes them predictable, while at the same time rendering them easy to engender and difficult to eradicate. Cohen goes on to explain this apparent conundrum. The causes of moral panics, he states, may appear to be a new phenomenon, but they are, in reality, 'camouflaged versions of traditional and well-known evils'. Although the factors causing the panic may indeed be dangerous or damaging in themselves, they are usually only a warning sign or a superficial representation of a more real and deeper danger or threat. Moreover, while both the cause of the panic and the panic itself may be very tangible and 'transparent', they are also 'opaque' as accredited experts must explain the perils behind the 'superficially harmless'.

Cohen (2002: viii–xxi) identifies seven familiar clusters of folk devils that engender the conditions of a moral panic: young, working-class, violent males; those who perpetrate school-based violence; people who use the wrong drugs in the wrong places; child abusers; sex offenders; welfare cheats and single mothers; and refugees and asylum seekers. It could be argued that we could add a further category of folk demon to this list: binge-drinking, violent, young white women.

In order for any particular social group to evoke a state of moral panic there must be a reaction to them. This reaction may have several different levels: concern; hostility; consensus; disproportionality; and volatility.

Hoodies tend to be a recent representation of the enduring young, working-class, violent male devils. The response to hoodies evident from some of the newspaper comments and the comments from young people themselves given above can range from concern and hostility to outright aggression and it does, to some degree, seem to be becoming a popular societal consensus.

Echoing Berger and Luckmann (1966), Cohen (2002) argues that the processes of demonization and the response to the demonized object add up to a socially constructed reality, and that in order for this new reality of devilish identity to take hold the response to and amplification of the response to anti-normative events needs to become embedded in the dominant cultural perspectives. A significant role in this response/amplification/embedding is played out through the broadcast and print media. However, as the next section of this chapter will show, other agencies of socialization also can play a part.

Case study: Philip becomes a devil in a hoodie

Earlier in this chapter, drawing on the work of Becker (1963), it was argued that identities can be socially constructed. This section will provide an illustration of this process through the case study of the demonization of a boy named Philip provided by Pollard, *et al.* (2000). Pollard, *et al.* (2000: 266) describe Philip as the youngest child of three from a supportive and stable family background whose mother was in employment, though his father was long-term unemployed. Philip was described by his teacher as 'always well-turned out, never scruffy or untidy, always well-mannered'.

Philip's school was in an area of extreme social disadvantage, with the highest take-up of free school meals in what was one of the poorest local authority areas in North West England. The school served a large overspill housing estate; there was a high level of male unemployment and many single parent families. A significant number of children attending Philip's school were 'at risk'. Throughout his primary school career, where mixed-aged classes were the norm, Philip's year group was described by his teachers as 'not as good' as the younger learners.

Pollard, *et al.* (2000) describe Year 4 as being pivotal in the creation of Philip's identity. In Year 3 his teacher described him as 'enjoying his work ... being responsive ... very much Mr Middle-of-the-Road' (ibid.: 267). Philip, up to this point, although being a low achiever and lacking confidence, was keen to do well. His work was neat, tidy and careful and he did not seem to have major problems with his work. By the end of Year 4, however, his teacher described him as 'extremely disruptive ... poor ability level ... confrontational ... difficult to handle ... a very tough little boy' (ibid). Philip had started to become aggressive to other children, and although he began to control this aggression in Year 5, his attitude to learning deteriorated. His Year 5 teacher described him as 'a pleasure to have' as long as he was not pressed to do any work. His lack of confidence in his ability appears to have become somewhat overwhelming. The teachers reported that if asked to write five sentences he would say: 'There's no way I'm going to be able to do that.'

By the time Philip was in Year 6, he appears to have completely disengaged with the learning process. His Year 6 teachers reported that most of the time he would sit and do very little work, moreover, if tackled about this he would sulk and refuse to do any more. During Year 6 Philip once again became aggressive, rude and surly, culminating in a direct challenge to authority in the swimming baths. When Philip's teachers tried to get him to see the error of his ways, his response was: 'I'm not bothered, don't care' (ibid.: 268). At the end of Key Stage 2 Philip achieved a Level 2 in maths and was ungraded in the SAT tests for English and science (although he was awarded a Level 2 in both on the basis of the tasks).

It would seem that Philip had enjoyed school up to the end of Year 3. He described Mr Matthews, his Year 3 teacher, as the 'best teacher in the world'. However, in Year 4 his teacher put him in the Red Group – those needing learning support and Philip became more and more aware of his own shortcomings: 'I just think I'm not any good – I always get stuck on some words.' Whereas in Year 3 Philip's teacher seemed keen to support him, this following quotation from his Year 4 teacher suggests a boy coming to terms with his new identity as a failure:

> He likes to be seen as tough … likes to mix with the tough ones in Year 5 …. He's a volcano … can't cope with the suggestion that he's in the wrong; tries to avoid it … he wants his own way … sulks … sometimes walks out of class.
>
> (ibid.: 269)

In Year 5 Philip was getting involved in fights in the playground and in bullying one younger, high-attaining boy in his class. However, when Philip did ask his Year 6 teacher for help in understanding a particular task the teacher said: 'There are plenty of others in the class who can't do it but they're not sulking' (ibid.: 271).

What this brief description of Philip's primary school life might suggest is how his sense of self as a learner was constructed and amplified through his interactions with his teachers. From here Philip would go on to become a bottom-set learner in his neighbourhood comprehensive school. His 'tough' identity led him towards associating with older boys at secondary school, on the edge of more and more 'trouble' until he became a fully fledged gang member, hanging around the shopping parade, constantly causing nuisance with shoppers and shopkeepers until being moved on by the police community support officer, and then coming to the attention of the local constable. Eventually labelled as a Persistent Young Offender, Philip wears his Anti-social Behaviour Order (ASBO) badge with pride and is the scourge of his local neighbourhood.

Although it is impossible to say for certain that Year 4 changed Philip's life, it does seem that the very different approaches that his Year 3 and his Year 4 teachers adopted towards his learning problems did have radical consequences for Philip. Thus it could be suggested that pupil–teacher interaction and teacher expectations of pupils are two of the most significant factors in a child's construction of their educational capabilities. In other words, these two factors are significant in a pupil's self-belief or self-efficacy in terms of educational achievement. When self-belief is limited and when this lack of self-belief is reinforced by low-level teacher expectations, 'self-handicapping strategies' (Mitchell 2004 cited in Matheson 2004: 88) such as disengagement from and rejection of the education system may come into place. Unfortunately, for children like Philip this may result in a rebellion against wider societal expectations and immersion in a counter-culture (see Willis 1978).

Activity 4.1.2: The fate of Philip

Having read the case study of Philip from Pollard, *et al.* (2000) given above, consider:
- What could have been done during Philip's primary-school education to prevent his disengagement with the education process?
- What could be done to help young people like Philip once they have reached secondary school, have disengaged with the education system and have been given an ASBO and/ or been labelled as a Persistent Young Offender?

Conclusion: devils or altar boys?

This chapter has highlighted the fact that the dominant reading of youths in hoodies is a negative one – a reading that has become normalized through media-driven narratives which create and feed moral panics in society. Nevertheless, other readings are possible.

When several shopping malls responded to the deviant image of youths in hoodies by banning young people wearing them – a move backed by the then Prime Minister Tony Blair (White and Dyer 2007) – David Cameron, leader of the Opposition expressed an alternative view. The *BBC News* website reported Cameron's suggestion that hoodies 'are more defensive than offensive', in the sense that wearing a hoodie may be a way, in a dangerous environment, to become invisible and blend in. In other words, wearing a hoodie is a response to a problem – the danger imminent in society – rather than the problem itself (Cameron cited by *BBC News* 2008). Moreover, in a deliberate attempt to destabilize the escalating construction of hoodies as devils, John Sentamu, Archbishop of York, was photographed wearing a hoodie in May 2008.

Youths wearing hoodies have been reported, among other positive activities, as having supported bullied youngsters through a peer mentoring programme at Longbenton Community College, Tyneside (*BBC Look North* 2008) and, at Lancaster and Morecambe College, supporting older people (*Lancaster Guardian* 2008). In a small way, these and other events help to redress the negative constructions being created about hoodies.

Furthermore, research has shown that there is a disproportionality to the negative narratives. Bagley, *et al.* (2009) report that less than 10 per cent of their sample of 1,450 young respondents in Manchester believed that people wearing hoodies were 'thugs or threatening', yet this response is the dominant mode of reporting.

Despite these positive interludes, the prevailing image of the youth in a hoodie is that of a devil or demon and, as such, as a valid cause of moral panic in society. As was suggested above, moral panics are volatile. While the object or source of moral panics shifts from time to time and from place to place, what does appear to remain constant, however, is the need for the public to panic and to construct a bogeyman on which to hang this panic. This is an interesting sociological and psychological phenomenon, which we have touched upon here and which is explored in detail elsewhere (cf. S. Cohen 1972; 1987; 2002).

Student reflection

Having read this chapter consider why hoodies have become a contemporary folk devil – why do you think they have become a demonized sector of society?

In conclusion, it is suggested here that the construction 'hoodies' creates, perpetuates and reinforces a false dualism – one that is strongly resistant to erosion. That dualism is an age-related dualism which writes adults and young people differently. Adults are the ones in a position to describe and inscribe young people as not yet complete, as adults-in-waiting, rather than as young people in their own right with their own identities (see Chapter 1.2, this volume). The discourses associated with this age-related dualism have a socially constructive and historically persistent trajectory and, as such, within the social mix that ascribes positive images and roles to some young people and negative images and roles to others. There has always been a dichotomic construction of children and youth and thus the demonization of hoodies is another manifestation of this. To save the hoodie we need to look at a much deeper level – at the language we use to construct children and young people.

Student reflection

The demonization of youth is in large part restricted to particular groups in our society largely based on characteristics such as class, ethnicity, and location. Why do you think these particular groups as seen as a threat to the adult world?

It might be useful to compare how these groups are viewed in other major industrial societies to see if the same process of demonization takes place and in the process reflect on what is happening with these societies. It might be useful to think about how this process relates to family structures, youth employment, educational failure, racism, urbanisation and poverty.

Key points

- Otherizing or demonizing of marginalized groups in society is not a new phenomenon.
- One of the groups who have been persistently demonized in the West is young, potentially violent males (S. Cohen 1972).
- This traditional folk devil has been reinvented as the hoodie, largely through media discourses.
- The effect of the media discourses has been so overwhelming that the construction of the hoodie has become a source of social and moral panic to such an extent that young people have become afraid of their own social group.
- In some parts of the country, in order to achieve official targets, police officers have pursued specific young people to such an extent that the young people have eventually been given ASBOs and/or been labelled as Persistent Young Offenders.
- It is suggested that teacher–pupil interactions and teacher expectations play a significant role in discouraging engagement with the education system and can pave the way for counter-culture behaviour and 'hoodyism'.
- The construction of the hoodie as a folk devil is a recent incarnation of the social age-related discourse of adults who write young people as incomplete and as adults in the making.
- In order to construct identities for children and young people in a more positive light we must examine how we use language and social discourses to create these identities.

Recommended reading

Becker, H. S. (1963) *Outsiders: Studies in the Sociology of Deviance*, New York: Free Press.

Cohen, S. (2002) *Folk Devils and Moral Panics: The Creation of the Mods and Rockers*, 3rd edn, London: Routledge.

Willis, P. (1978) *Learning to Labour: How Working Class Kids Get Working Class Jobs*, London: Saxon House.

References

Bagley, K., Davies, C., Harris, J. and Robinson, J. (2009) *The Children and Young People's Plan: Advice to Manchester Children's Services Authority*, Manchester: MHM/CUE.

Bartlett, R. (2008) Speaking to *The Radio Times*, in Clout (2008).

Bawdon, F (2009) *Hoodies or Altar Boys? what is media stereotyping doing to our British boys?* Women in Journalism/Echo Research, London. Available online at: http://www.womeninjournalism. co.uk/node/325 (accessed 18.03.2009).

BBC News (2008) Cameron to make 'hoodie' appeal. Available online at: http://news.bbc.co.uk/1/ hi/uk_politics/5162010.stm (accessed 09.03.2009).

BBC Look North (2008) Hoodies tackle bullying through peer mentoring. Available online at: http://www.mandbf.org.uk/news/newsinfo/article/3675/40/ (accessed 09.03.2009).

Becker, H. S. (1963) *Outsiders: Studies in the Sociology of Deviance*, New York: Free Press.

Berger, P. and Luckmann, T. (1966) *The Social Construction of Reality: A Treatise in the Sociology of Knowledge*, New York/Harmondsworth: Anchor Books/Penguin Books.

Byron, T. (2009) We see children as pestilent, *Education Guardian*, 17 March: 1–2.

Carroll, S (2009) Enforced conscription is the answer to sick yobs, *Daily Mirror*, 2 March. Cited in: Bawdon, F. (2009) *Hoodies or Altar Boys? what is media stereotyping doing to our British boys?* Women in Journalism/Echo Research, London. Available online at: http://www.womeninjournalism.co.uk/ node/325 (accessed 18.03.2009).

Clout, L. (2008) 'Hoodies' were the scourge of Medieval London, *Telegraph*, 8 April. Available online at: http://www.telegraph.co.uk/news/uknews/1584317/Hoodies-were-the-scourge-of-Medieval-London.html (accessed 09.03.2009).

Cohen, A. K. (1955) *Delinquent Boys: The Culture of the Gang*, Chicago: Free Press.

Cohen, P. (1972) Subcultural conflict and working class community, *Working Papers in Cultural Studies*, 2: 5–52.

Cohen, S. (1972) *Folk Devils and Moral Panics: The Creation of the Mods and Rockers*, 1st edn, London: MacGibbon and Kee Ltd.

—— (1987) *Folk Devils and Moral Panics: The Creation of the Mods and Rockers*, 2nd edn, Oxford: Basil Blackwell Ltd.

—— (2002) *Folk Devils and Moral Panics: The Creation of the Mods and Rockers*, 3rd edn, London: Routledge.

Corrigan, P. (1979) *Schooling the Smash Street Kids*, London: Macmillan.

Engaging Communities Foundation (2006) *2020 Every Child in Bolton Matters: Report of Bolton's CSA Future Search*, Bolton: ECF.

Garner, R. (2009) 'Hoodies, louts, scum': how media demonises teenagers, *Independent*, 13 March. Available online at: http://www.independent.co.uk/news/uk/home-news/hoodies-louts-scum-how-media-demonizes-teenagers-1643964.html (accessed 18.03.2009).

Giddens, A. (1979) *Central Problems in Social Theory*, Basingstoke: Macmillan.

Hall, S. and Jefferson, T. (eds) (1976) *Resistance Through Ritual: Youth Subcultures in Post-war Britain*, London: Hutchinson.

Hebdige, D. (1979) *Subculture: The Meaning of Style*, London: Methuen.

Lancaster Guardian (2008) Hoodies help out OAPs, *Lancaster Guardian*. Available online at: http:// www.lancasterguardian.co.uk/lancasternews/Hoodies-help-out-OAPs.5020886.jp (accessed 09.03.2009).

Littlejohn, R. (2008) Nobody calls the Boy Scouts 'animals', rants Barnardo's boss, *Daily Mail*, 18 November. Cited in: Bawdon, F. (2009) *Hoodies or Altar Boys? what is media stereotyping doing to our British boys?* Women in Journalism/Echo Research, London. Available online at: http:// www.womeninjournalism.co.uk/node/325 (accessed 18.03.2009).

Matheson, D. (ed.) *An Introduction to the Study of Education*, 2nd edn, London: David Fulton Publishers Ltd.

Mitchell, G. (2004) Psychology in education, in D. Matheson (ed.) *An Introduction to the Study of Education*, 2nd edn, London: David Fulton Publishers Ltd.

Moore, S. (2009) We demonise all boys as feral … then wonder why they turn into hoodies, *Mail Online*, 14 March. Available online at: http://www.mailonsunday.co.uk/debate/article-1162026/ SUZANNE-MOORE-We-demonise-boys-feral---wonder-turn-hoodies.html (accessed 18.09.2009).

Newman, S. (2007) 'Wags' and 'hoodies' included in new dictionary, *Independent*. Available online at: http://www.independent.co.uk/news/uk/this-britain/wags-and-hoodies-included-in-new-dictionary-451676.html (accessed 09.03.2009).

Pollard, A., Triggs, P., Broadfoot, P., McNess, E. and Osborn, M. (2000) *What Pupils Say: Changing Policy and Practice in Primary Education – Findings from the PACE Project*, London: Continuum.

The Insider (2009) Cashing in on hoodies, Channel 4, 16 February. Available online at: http://www.channel4.com/news/articles/ontv/theinsider/cashing+in+on+the+hoodies/570037 (accessed 09.03.2009).

White, J. and Dyer, L. (2007) Hoodie hoodlums: loved or loathed?, Headliners. Available online at: http://www.headliners.org/storylibrary/stories/2005/hoodiehoodlumsloveorloathed.htm (accessed 09.03.2009).

Willis, P. (1978) *Learning to Labour: How Working Class Kids Get Working Class Jobs*, London: Saxon House.

4.2 The testing regime of childhood

Up against the wall

Terry Wrigley

Assessement and power

Knowledge is always entangled with power (Foucault 1977), but especially so when we exercise the authority to make judgements about other people. And of course, adults are constantly making judgements about children. From a very early age, we tell them they are good or naughty, we praise them for being strong or clever, we approve and disapprove. These judgements can be more or less benign, but they invariably serve to mould children, to a degree, into the hegemonic norms of the contemporary adult society.

School assessment represents a particularly public and authoritative mode of evaluation. The teacher and the school system, on behalf of society, make judgements about a young person's acquisition of knowledge and their whole development which claim a high degree of objectivity. The judgements are shared with the learner but also with others in authority, within and beyond the school. They are formally recorded in ways which have an enduring impact. Many forms of assessment produce labels which impact psychologically on young people, and which serve as keys and locks to open or close potential futures.

Assessment is not just the articulation of knowledge about another, it is the assertion and exercise of power. Some of this is explicit, but, like other ways in which power is exercised, there is often a self-concealment. This does not in the slightest diminish the power; rather it can exacerbate it: 'Power is at its most effective when least observable' (Lukes 2005: 1).

In terms of school assessment, the criteria underlying judgements may be hidden, and unreliability or even bias can be concealed. Beyond this, however, there is a silence around the power structures and value systems of the wider society which has helped to shape and will use the assessments: the assessment act appears discrete and limited and without imbrication in wider social structures and value systems. One aim of this chapter is to uncover these connections.

School assessment can, of course, take many different forms, some more benign than others, but is unavoidably entangled with power. Assessment regimes are also regimes of truth-power. It is better for us to articulate and argue this entanglement than to pretend it isn't there, since we can only act to change them if we understand how they operate and whose interests they may be serving.

'Truth' is to be understood as a system of ordered procedures for the production, regulation, distribution, circulation, and operation of statements. 'Truth' is linked in a circular relation with systems of power which produce and sustain it, and to effects of power which it induces and which extends it – a 'regime' of truth .... It's not a matter of emancipating truth from every system of power (which would be a chimera, for truth is already power), but of detaching the power of truth from the forms of hegemony, social, economic and cultural, within which it operates at the present time.

(Foucault 2002: 132–3)

A particular focus of this chapter is to examine the regimes of high-stakes testing established in the most powerful English-speaking countries in recent decades, and which have had varying levels of influence elsewhere. It will however set this in context by examining some previous assessment regimes. Finally, it will explore some alternatives for their educational and social advantages.

Assessment and modernity

It is too easy to regard the forms of assessment to which we are accustomed as a permanent and universal feature of education systems. Historical comparisons help us to relativize and see beyond contemporary norms.

To take a simple example, there is an assumption in English-speaking countries that a written examination is the appropriate guarantor of satisfactory completion of university studies, yet the medieval custom of orally defending your arguments remains paramount in much of continental Europe. It is assumed across Britain that examinations are necessary to ensure suitability for university studies, yet in nineteenth-century Scotland attendance at university lectures was not dependent on a qualifying examination, thus creating relatively easy access to higher education for people of different social classes (Anderson 1989).

Foucault's remarkable *Discipline and Punish* (1991) traces some of the early manifestations of 'examination' and its impact on modern life. Relating disciplinary regimes of various kinds (prisons, military, schools, hospitals), he highlights a change of practice from the rare display of knowledge (e.g. the master-work at the end of a guild apprenticeship) to regular testing.

> The Brothers of the Christian Schools wanted their pupils to be examined every day of the week: on the first for spelling, on the second for arithmetic, on the third for catechism in the morning and for handwriting in the afternoon, etc. Moreover, there was to be an examination each month in order to pick out those who deserved to be submitted for examination by the inspector.
>
> (Foucault 1991: 186)

Foucault argues that this regime of testing 'combines the techniques of an observing hierarchy and those of a normalizing judgement. It is a normalizing gaze, a surveillance that makes it possible to qualify, to classify and to punish' (ibid.: 184). It is a technology of individualization, making each individual a 'case' to be 'described, judged, measured, compared with others, in his very individuality; and it is also the individual who has to be trained or corrected, classified, normalized, excluded etc.' (ibid: 191). And this was part of a wider disciplining – of activity, of time, of relationships – which helped create a culture of factory work and modern state bureaucracies.

This disciplinary individualization, again too easily taken for granted, is deeply at odds with a Vygotskian understanding of learning as the socio-cultural construction of knowledge (Vygotsky 1986, 1978; Salomon 1993; Perkins 1992). It also runs counter to the informal emancipatory learning which happens wherever people combine to struggle for their rights and for a better future (e.g. trade unions, social movements).

This is not to suggest that individual examinations are always harmful or can easily be dispensed with. Historically, an entrance examination for entry to the civil service helped to overcome a system of patronage. Likewise, few of us would want to be treated by a doctor whose knowledge had not been carefully checked – though it is important to acknowledge that the interpersonal skills and the instinctive hunches which real-life diagnosis involves cannot be tested in the same way.

New assessment regimes rarely achieve dominance just as technical innovations. The introduction of mass publicly-funded elementary education in late-Victorian Britain was accompanied by regular in-class testing and periodic verification by visiting inspectors, and the school's budget depended upon this: 'Payment by Results'. This was justified in terms of economy not quality: 'if it is not cheap it shall be efficient; if it is not efficient it shall be cheap' (Robert Lowe, quoted in Lawson and Silver 1973: 290). This encouraged rote-learning and a narrowing down and debasement of the curriculum; less testable skills and understandings were neglected. As T. H. Huxley later put it: 'The Revised Code did not compel any schoolmaster to leave off teaching anything; but, by the very simple process of refusing to pay for many kinds of teaching, it practically put an end to them' (ibid: 290–1).

It also led to a debased and instrumental relationship with children, and a neglect of those children who did not score well:

> Edward Thring looked back at the experience of payment by results and the inspection of minds like 'specimens on a board with a pin stuck through them like beetles', and appealed to teachers to get rid of the vestiges of the system: 'strive for liberty to teach, have mercy on the slow, the ignorant, the weak'.
>
> (ibid: 292)

These judgements are equally applicable to current systems of 'high-stakes testing' (see below).

The first half of the twentieth century was dominated by a new testing regime, which served as the gatekeeper for secondary education. The notion of a 'general intelligence', assumed to be largely innate, allowed only a tiny minority of working-class pupils access to secondary schools.

There is not the time here to critique the concept of innate general intelligence ('IQ') or its assessment (see for example Wrigley 2003: 75–90). It is important however to recognize the social and political circumstances in which this became the dominant orthodoxy. In Victorian times, it was normal to speak openly of preparing boys and girls 'for their station in life', namely the same occupational levels as their parents; reference to the general intellectual inferiority of the 'lower orders' was normal in the discourse of that era. Such blatant upper class attitudes became impossible with the rise of the labour movement (trade unions, the early Labour Party); a new discourse was required which would justify the exclusion of most working-class children from higher levels of education on the grounds of their meagre 'intelligence'.

Faced with such increasing radical activity, the language of class arrogance was hardly appropriate .... It was becoming no longer possible to dismiss the vast majority of working class children as being unfit to receive a secondary education because of their class alone.

(Cowburn 1986: 122–5)

At roughly the same time, the skills shortage following the loss of life in the First World War necessitated allowing a minority of higher-attaining working-class children into grammar schools. Thus the 11-plus exam or 'scholarship' became the mechanism where a few could be granted grammar school places free of charge while labelling the rest as intellectually incapable. (It should be noted, however, that many still didn't make it, despite passing the '11-plus'; their parents couldn't afford the school uniform!)

Testing for this mysterious essence of 'intelligence' had a doubly ideological function: it appeared to justify the social hierarchy by appeal to the 'science' of psychological testing while loading many workers with a lifelong sense that they were incapable of more complex learning and that they should leave the thinking to others. It perpetuated the Victorian view that society divided naturally into hands and brains.

The long-term damage this caused to Britain's cultural and economic development later became apparent with the founding of comprehensive schools, and the sudden upsurge of examination success and university entrance among those who had previously been thought ineducable (Tomlinson 2004: 63).

The age of high-stakes testing

Assessment is centrally concerned with evaluating learning and acting upon that evaluation. It can have a range of functions, such as feedback, diagnosis, confirming the acquisition of knowledge and allocating learners into different courses and institutions for further study.

The term *high-stakes testing* was coined, originally in the USA, to designate assessment which has additional and serious consequences. This usefully describes the assessment regime which was established in the UK (England in particular) during the 1990s, and which continues until the present. (The term could also be applied retrospectively to the 'payment by results' of the Revised Code – see above.)

The emergence of high-stakes testing around 1990 can only be understood within the context of marketized schooling. Indeed, it was introduced deliberately to create the conditions for an education market. The ideologues of the Thatcher government believed that the best form of regulation, and the best way to improve attainment, was for individual schools to rise or fall in a competitive market. Schools with lower exam and test results would attract fewer students, and be forced to close because their budget became unmanageable. The pupils would move to neighbouring schools who would build additional accommodation, or a new school would open on the site of the failing school. The mechanism would be parental choice, stimulated by league-table presentations of test scores. In effect, the state devised an assessment regime in order to create and stimulate a quasi-market.

This neglected many factors. Better educated or more ambitious parents became adept at avoiding lower-attaining schools, leaving behind a residue of families without the material or cultural resources to make a choice. In many urban areas, less attractive schools became concentrations of poverty and disadvantage, a problem exacerbated by them having to take in pupils excluded by their more successful competitors. In effect the system created, rather than identified, 'failing schools'.

These processes were exacerbated by a system of full-spectrum surveillance: teacher appraisal, a hostile inspection regime, performance pay and so on. The system invented by a Conservative government was sustained by New Labour, but with a new edge to it: the rush to hand over publicly funded schools into private management. The City Academies project was invented (see http://www.antiacademies.org.uk; Beckett 2007). Ostensibly to deal with the problem of 'failing schools', it is now easier to see the real issue as a desire to privatize public services (an aspect of neoliberalism). Not only was school 'failure' generated by a competitive market system, the government also keeps raising the height of the hurdles which schools are required to jump. In the spring of 2008, under the euphemism of a 'National Challenge', all secondary schools with fewer than 30 per cent of pupils gaining five or more A*–C grades including English and mathematics were threatened with closure. This meant one in five secondary schools.

Two-thirds of schools where more than a third of pupils had a free-meal entitlement were deemed failing. This would lead a more self-critical government to ask itself whether perhaps its own policies for inner-city and council-estate schools had failed, rather than the schools. (Ironically, the 'failures' included schools which had already been privatized – 26 academies. Would these be returned to local authority control?)

A similar pattern has been ruthlessly pursued on the other side of the Atlantic. The USA's high-stakes regime, misleadingly known as No Child Left Behind (NCLB), constantly raises the hurdle, making it impossible for many schools to succeed, until publicly funded schools are handed over to private businesses (Hursh 2007; Lipman 2007).

Besides the drama of privatization and asset-stripping, a high-stakes assessment regime has many other side effects.

- *A narrower curriculum.* It leads teachers (and pupils) to focus only on what is tested. This can involve much time spent on practice tests; neglecting other subjects such as history or music; or concentrating on a narrow range of skills within language and mathematics. Sometimes this narrowing is reinforced by curriculum directives, e.g. the promotion of a narrow view of 'reading' as merely decoding the letters (phonics). Resources are diverted from other educational goals and activities:

  > For example, McNeil reports that a low-scoring school serving primarily Mexican-American students had no library, a shortage of texts and little laboratory equipment, yet administrators spent $20,000 for commercial test-preparation books.
  >
  > (Lipman 2008: 43)

- *Privileging some pupils while neglecting others.* When a hurdle is set such as 'the percentage of pupils reaching level 4 at age 11', or 'the percentage with five A*–Cs at age 16', schools are led to concentrate on those pupils who are nearly there. (The US term is 'bubble kids': see Booher-Jennings 2005; Neal and Schanzenbach 2007; Lipman 2004: 43). The process has been described as *triage* – like hospital emergency units which divide patients into beyond recovery, trivial injuries, and priorities for attention. Giving the Ds extra attention to turn them into Cs can lead to the appearance of rapid school improvement, but it sidelines the needs of the rest to achieve their potential.

- *Deterring teachers from more troubled schools.* There have always been reasons why many teachers wish to avoid schools in high-poverty neighbourhoods, but the mechanisms of performance pay and hostile inspection exacerbate this. Teachers are led to fear that they will put their careers at risk by teaching in the schools that need them most.
- *An instrumental attitude towards young people.* A high-stakes testing regime exerts a steady, subtle and sometimes overwhelming pressure on teachers to see their pupils as levels rather than children.

> How many teachers, particularly those of younger children, are now able to listen openly, attentively, and in a non-instrumental, exploratory way to their children/ students without feeling guilty, stressed or vaguely uncomfortable about about the absence of criteria or the insistence of a target tugging at their sleeves.
>
> (Fielding 1999: 280)

It is impossible to prove that the assessment regime has led to an erosion of humane and caring relationships, and contributed substantially to the unhappiness and instability of a generation of young people, but there is a case to answer (Hursh 2007).

- *Self-deceit at the highest level.* Eventually politicians are themselves caught in the snares of high-stakes systems and the promises that they will lead to higher standards. A government target was set of 80 per cent of 11-year-olds reaching level 4 in reading, with the education minister promising he would resign if it wasn't reached; the tests were immediately made easier to ensure that it would be (Hilton 2001; Tymms 2004). The new reading tests reduced the number of questions requiring inference and evaluation as opposed to straightforward recognition of facts. A similar fix occurred at age 16. Here the key benchmark was the percentage of pupils in a school achieving five or more A*–C grades: an easier GNVQ certificate was then redefined as 'equivalent' to four A*–C grades, such that pupils only needed this and one other GCSE. Sadly, although politicians might assert that 1 and 1 makes 5, the young people themselves were unlikely to be able to use this credential as a passport into higher levels of education or well paying careers. The exact reasons for this sleight of hand are still obscure, but it may have been devised to create the illusion that the government's policies were helping urban schools in deprived neighbourhoods (see also Haney 2000 for the 'Texas miracle').

The ideological impact of high-stakes testing

A high-stakes regime does also work ideologically – like the IQ tests of the early twentieth century (see above), but on an institutional as well as individual scale. It takes public attention away from the intolerably high levels of poverty in places like Britain and the USA, placing the blame on schools for not being 'effective'.

The fermenting of moral panics around educational 'failure' (real, exaggerated or imagined) is now documented in a number of education systems (e.g. Lipman 2004: 2 for the USA; Sears 2003 for Canada).

> On 12 September 1995, the first Education Minister in Ontario's Conservative government told education officials that 'If we really want to fundamentally change the issue in training and ... education we'll have to first make sure we've communicated brilliantly the breakdown in the process we currently experience. That's not

easy. We need to invent a crisis. That's not just an act of courage. There's some skill involved.'

(Sears 2003: 3–4)

In the USA, the launching of Sputnik by the Soviet Union ahead of America's space programme led to a panic about problems in the school system; the connection was spurious, but so too were the 'school effectiveness' strategies that emerged. It led to an increase in drilling learners and transmission pedagogies, a denigration of progressive school reform and neglect of critical thinking, as well as the promulgation of 'teacher-proof' curriculum packages. In Britain, Margaret Thatcher fought an election campaign with the slogan 'Education isn't working'. Ever since, state schools have been blamed for poverty, the state of the economy, social breakdown and moral decline.

Culture, identities and social justice

It is tempting to see testing as the root cause of problems in our education system, and the current assessment regime does act as the motor which drives much of the rest. However the prime locus for understanding the multiple connections lies further back, in the economic and political configuration known as neoliberalism.

Neoliberalism has fittingly been described as 'capitalism with the gloves off'. It is an attempt to return to days of raw capitalism untempered by social security and the welfare state. Originally understood and promoted as 'market rather than state', neoliberalism uses both in tandem: the state is used to create markets, as well as for more overt exercises of power (policing and imperial conquest), while more benign 'welfare state' functions are marginalized. As David Harvey (2005) and others have demonstrated, the core purpose is to increase exploitation and the profit of the super-rich, rather than any ideological anti-statism.

It is also too easy to blame 'middle-class' parents for an obsession with results. The term is quite misleading, as it consists, in the majority, of white-collar and professional workers who are also exploited in an economic system run for the benefit of the super-rich. The growth of neoliberalism, including a finance system which relies on high levels of debt (now revealed as perilously fragile) and the loss of job security, encourages 'middle-class' as well as manual worker families to try to safeguard their children's futures in a situation which has been made precarious and competitive.

Neoliberalism's declared preference for hands-off management can go hand-in-hand with more draconian exercise of central state power. In the education system, the Thatcher government simultaneously 'freed' school management from local authorities while tightening central government control through a standardized National Curriculum, high-stakes testing and inspection. Schools and particularly head teachers gained control over their own budgets but crucially lost control over what was taught. This was reinforced under New Labour through increasing central control over the details of how teaching would happen (the various Strategies).

Test results were presented as a natural calibrator for schools' 'accountability' to parents. It is right and proper that teachers accept a responsibility to parents and society as a whole, but that is different from the current level of politically stimulated anxiety: '"Accountability" is, after all, not the same thing as responsibility, still less duty. It is a pistol loaded with blame to be fired at the heads of those who cannot answer charges' (Inglis 1989: 35–54).

Accountability through testing is highly reductionist in terms of the information which is communicated between teachers, parents and young people. It forms part of the regime of truth which Nikolas Rose calls 'government by numbers' (Rose 1999). The problem of reductionism is important not only in terms of information transmitted, but also in terms of discourse and action. It normalizes particular ways of speaking about young people and education. It also leads to some activities being prioritized and others marginalized. In schools, we have seen many parallels to the bean-counting imposed on the police: targets for the number of arrests have led police to pursue petty offences while neglecting more serious ones which take longer to solve. It results in crude evaluation and policy development – rather like Stalinist Russia where increasing the tonnage of pig-iron production stood as a proxy for socially responsible economic development.

Within such a regime, attempts to make allowances for poverty and social inequality too easily collapse or produce a distorted understanding. School effectiveness theory in Britain has used free school meal (FSM) entitlement as a means of moderating crude comparison by test scores, largely because these were the most easily available data. Schools were compared against 'similar' schools (according to FSM) and charged with having lower than expected proportions gaining five A*–Cs. The FSM measure was not only crude, it was deeply illogical: it completely fails to look at how many pupils in each school have the kind of financial or educational advantages which would facilitate them achieving these higher qualifications. My own analysis (as yet unpublished) of Scottish data has shown a very close correlation (far higher than FSM) between the proportion of pupils achieving three or more highers (essential for university entry) and the proportion with graduate mothers. And ultimately, governments are quite prepared to drop all pretence at benchmarking. Gordon Brown's ministers made no allowance whatsoever for socio-economic disadvantage when labelling all schools as failing where fewer than 30 per cent gained five A*–Cs with English and maths (the 'National Challenge', see above).

At an individual level too, the testing regime has failed to improve social justice. Though intelligent assessment is important in order to monitor progress, diagnose difficulties and identify pupils in need of additional support – especially among sections of the population most at risk – high-stakes testing within a competitive quasi-market environment appears to have the opposite effect. High-pressure test-preparation is a poor substitute for engaging pupils' enthusiasm and interest, and soon proves unsustainable. The testing regime has also led to forms of labelling and segregation from an early age: those children who are placed on the tortoise table at age six rarely move groups to become hares.

Government by numbers also operates across national boundaries. The OECD (a powerful engine which predominantly operates, alongside the World Bank and IMF, to foster capitalist forms of economic development) runs the PISA international tests. The tests themselves are of good quality, and data analysis has highlighted important issues of injustice. (Examples include the adverse impact of Germany's selective system, see Baumert and Schümer (2002); and the differential impact of growing up in single-parent families in countries with differing welfare provision, see Haahr *et al.* (2005: 88).)

However, the comparisons can also be used by politicians to engender a climate of intimidation in order to promote reactionary school reforms. Thus, Norway's Conservative education minister declared it shameful that their schools were 'only average', and introduced national tests linked to inter-school competition, quasi-markets, and privately managed schools. Her reforms collapsed (as did her government within a few years) because of a widespread boycott by 15-year-olds: a quarter handed in blank sheets of paper on the recommendations of the *elevorganisasjon* (pupil union). International tests such as PISA, focusing on language (i.e. the national language), maths and science, take no account of cultural or curricular differences. For example, Norway's 15-year-olds are required to write accurately *both* official versions of Norwegian, to be fluent in English, and (most of them) to begin another European language. PISA takes no account of the time this takes. Similarly, it gives no credit for the strong environmental emphasis of Norway's schools, the quality of care and social relationships, and the initiative and responsibility developed through inter-disciplinary projects.

To base policy change on crude comparisons and competition leads to a speeding up of the educational conveyor belt, rather than real qualitative improvements or carefully considered school transformation: 'What really matters: new targets to meet? higher maths grades perhaps? or caring and creative learners, a future, a sense of justice, the welfare of the planet and its people?' (Wrigley 2003: 7).

Activity 4.2.1: Testing, politics and justice

Having read the above, explain, in your own words, how testing is related to politics and social justice.

Alternatives

The development of high-stakes systems from the early 1990s in Britain rested on a finding of school effectiveness research that assessment was a contributory factor towards schools helping their pupils achieve higher. This was based on a superficial reading. The classic *School Matters* study of inner-London primary schools (Mortimore, *et al.* 1988) distinguished between (a) schools whose teachers passed on information from year to year, whether in the form of grades or in the form of portfolios of work, from (b) schools where no information was passed on. The real issue is ensuring continuity and progress.

Many experts and educators placed some faith in the system devised around the National Curriculum. They appreciated its criterion-referencing (i.e. descriptors of what pupils could do) as a replacement for an earlier emphasis on norm-referencing (e.g. rank order within the class, or abstract numerical or lettered grades), though unfortunately the ladders of criteria turned into a new kind of competitive labelling, a new blend of norm- and criterion-referencing in which an overall amalgamated 'level' obscured specific strengths and weaknesses. Most teachers were, however, from the start suspicious of the over-reliance on externally-set and marked written tests, as opposed to teacher assessment. (Scotland avoided having all children sit down for a common test on the one day; instead teachers set an appropriate level of test when they felt particular children were ready, to verify their own judgement. This was however undermined in many authorities by pressure to show maximum progress each school year. Now England has adopted the Scottish system, but the same negative pressures may well occur.)

Over the years, pressure has built up for an alternative. There were successful boycotts between 1990 and 1995, though other unions failed to unite with the NUT. (The government managed to appease the NASUWT, more concerned about workload than the educational damage, by employing external markers.) Despite active campaigning by the Anti-SATs Alliance, founded in 2003, and an NUT boycott ballot in the same year (over 80 per cent in favour, but too low a turnout to implement), the system has not yet been abolished. It has however been considerably weakened, including the final abolition of Key Stage 3 SATs in 2008 following the disastrous failure of that summer's tests which had been contracted and out-sourced to a large commercial company in the USA.

Experts such as Paul Black who had earlier worked with the government to develop scales of levels for the National Curriculum campaigned forcefully for *formative assessment* (Assessment for Learning). Their research had demonstrated the importance of clear feedback to pupils, as opposed to summative grading. Unfortunately, though this has strong popular as well as official support, it is expected to operate in tandem with high-stakes summative testing and within a competitive environment.

Another important initiative, though little known in Britain, is the notion of *authentic assessment*. Newman and Archbald (1992) argue that assessment should where possible be integral to learning, and that assessment tasks should be educationally worthwhile, as learning experiences, in themselves in order not to create a diversion or distortion. Their idea was adopted in Queensland, Australia, under the name 'rich tasks' (now, in a more flexible form, known as 'blueprints'), and are beginning to be adopted and piloted by Scottish education authority Argyle and Bute in the context of Scotland's curriculum reform, *A Curriculum for Excellence*.

Rich tasks have to be valuable in themselves and not distract from real learning. They culminate in individual or team presentations, based on research and problem solving. They involve a range of skills, often connecting different subjects. The challenge must be meaningful to the learners – it could be set in a local context, with the results presented to an audience of parents or a community group.

Examples of rich tasks

*   *Multimedia presentation of an endangered plant or animal.* Students will investigate a threatened species and the extent to which it is at risk. They will use this investigation to take constructive action and create a persuasive and informative multimedia presentation.
*   *National identity: influences and perspectives.* This project involves the planning, production and presentation of a filmed documentary including information gleaned from research and interviews with people from different cultural backgrounds.
*   *The shape we're in.* Students investigate alternative shapes and/or dimensions for at least one container, a domestic object, a mechanical device and an object from nature. They then present an alternative design, explaining the maths.
*   *Opinion-making oracy.* Students will make forceful speeches on an issue of international or national significance to different audiences.

Conclusion

If we really want to improve educational standards, we should use assessment that enhances learning rather than trivializing it. We need to promote assessment which helps to develop co-operation and the building of learning communities, and which will re-engage young people who are often alienated and demoralized by the present assessment regime.

Student reflection

Consider the examples of 'rich tasks' given above.

*   Do you think they are a valid alternative to traditional tests?

Key points

*   Assessments may appear to be objective but are judgemental and entangled with power. Foucault (1991: 184) argues that assessments are a 'normalizing judgement'.
*   Many forms of assessment produce labels which can impact psychologically on young people and affect their futures, such as access to secondary or higher education.
*   The impact of assessments can be traced historically, such as the Victorian 'payment by results' and the narrowing of the curriculum, through the 11-plus exam and restricted access to grammar schools, to the current high-stakes testing.
*   Assessment should be concerned with evaluating learning and acting upon that evaluation. High-stakes testing was named to define assessment which has additional and serious consequences.
*   High-stakes testing is linked to marketized schooling and payment by results. Lower exam and test results, resulting in published league tables, can mean fewer students and a lower budget or even closure of schools.
*   It can be argued that high-stakes testing can lead to a narrowed curriculum, the unfair treatment of pupils, a lack of teachers for 'troubled' schools, an instrumental attitude to young people, and self-deceit by the government.
*   Ideologically, high-stakes testing places the blame on schools for not being 'effective' rather than examining the impact of social issues such as poverty upon the education process and therefore does not improve social justice.
*   Alternatives to testing highlight the importance of formative assessment involving teacher feedback on the processes and results of learning, e.g. 'Assessment for Learning'; and authentic assessment involving 'rich tasks' which are valuable in their own right and enhance rather than distort learning.

Recommended reading

Foucault, M. (2002) *Essential Works of Foucault 1954–84 vol. 3*, J. Faubion (ed.), London: Penguin.

Lipman, P. (2004) *High Stakes Education: Inequality, Globalization, and Urban School Reform*, New York: RoutledgeFalmer.

Ross, W. and Gibson, R. (2007) (eds) *Neoliberalism and Education Reform*, Creskill, NJ: Hampton Press.

Wrigley, T. (2003) *Schools of Hope: A New Agenda for School Improvement*, Stoke-on-Trent: Trentham.

References

Anderson, R. D. (1989) *Education and Opportunity in Victorian Scotland*, Edinburgh: Edinburgh UP.

Baumert, J. and Schümer, G. (2002) Family background, selection and achievement: the German experience, *Improving Schools* 5 (3): 13–20.

Beckett, F. (2007) *The Great City Academy Fraud*, London: Continuum.

Benn, M. and Chitty, C. (eds) *A Tribute to Caroline Benn: Education and Democracy*, London: Continuum.

Berlak, H., Newman, F. M., Adams, E., Archbald, D. A., Burgess, T., Raven, J. and Romberg, T. A. *Toward a New Science of Educational Testing and Assessment*, New York: SUNY.

Booher-Jennings, J. (2005) Below the bubble: 'educational triage' and the Texas accountability system, *American Educational Research Journal*, 42 (2): 231–68.

Cowburn, W. (1986) *Class, Ideology and Community Education*, London: Croom Helm.

Fielding, M. (1999) Target setting, policy pathology and student perspectives: learning to labour in new times, *Cambridge Journal of Education*, 29 (2): 277–87.

Foucault, M. (1977) *Power/Knowledge: Selected Interviews and Other Writings 1972–1977*, New York: Pantheon.

—— (1991) *Discipline and Punish: The Birth of the Prison*, London: Penguin.

—— (2002) *Essential Works of Foucault 1954–1984 vol. 3*, J. Faubion (ed.), London: Penguin.

Haahr, J., Nielsen, T. K., Hansen, M. E. and Jakobsen, S. T. (2005) *Explaining Student Performance: Evidence from the International PISA, TIMSS and PIRLS Survey*, Brussels: Danish Technological Institute. Available online at http://www.pisa.oecd.org/dataoecd/5/45/35920726.pdf (accessed 31.10.08).

Haney, W. (2000) The myth of the Texas Miracle in education, *Education Policy Analysis Archives*, 8 (41).

Harvey, D. (2005) *A Brief History of Neoliberalism*, Oxford: Oxford University Press.

Hilton, M. (2001) Are the key stage 2 reading tests becoming easier each year? *Reading*, 35 (1): 4–11.

Hursh, D. W. (2007) Neoliberalism and the control of teachers, students and learning: the rise of standards, standardization and accountability, in W. Ross and R. Gibson (eds) *Neoliberalism and Education Reform*, Creskill, NJ: Hampton Press.

Inglis, F. (1989) Managerialism and morality, in W. Carr (ed.) *Quality in Teaching: Arguments for a Reflective Professional*, London: Falmer.

Lawson, J. and Silver, H. (1973) *A Social History of Education in England*, London: Methuen.

Lipman, P. (2004) *High Stakes Education: Inequality, Globalization, and Urban School Reform*, New York: RoutledgeFalmer.

—— (2007) No Child Left Behind: globalization and the politics of race, in W. Ross and R. Gibson (eds) *Neoliberalism and Education Reform*, Creskill NJ: Hampton Press.

Lukes, S. (2005) *Power – A Radical View*, 2nd edn, Basingstoke: Palgrave Macmillan.

Mortimore, P., Sammons, P., Stoll, L., Lewis, D. and Ecob, R. (1988) *School Matters: The Junior Years*, Wells, Somerset: Open Books.

Neal, D. and Schanzenbach, D. (2007) *Left Behind by Design: Proficiency Counts and Test-based Accountability*, NBER Working Paper No. 13293. Available online at: http://home.uchicago.edu/%7En9na/web_ver_final.pdf (accessed 31.10.08).

Newman F. and Archbald, D. (1992) The nature of authentic academic achievement, in H. Berlak, F. M. Newman, E. Adams, D. A. Archbald, T. Burgess, J. Raven and T.A. Romberg (eds) *Toward a New Science of Educational Testing and Assessment*, New York: SUNY.

Perkins, D. (1992) *Smart Schools: Better Thinking and Learning for Every Child*, New York: The Free Press.

Rose, N. (1999) *Powers Of Freedom: Reframing Political Thought*, Cambridge: Cambridge University Press.

Ross, E. W. and Gibson, R. (2007) (eds) *Neoliberalism and Education Reform*, Creskill, NJ: Hampton Press.

Salomon, G. (1993) (ed.) *Distributed Cognitions: Psychological and Educational Considerations*, Cambridge: Cambridge University Press.

Sears, A. (2003) *Retooling the Mind Factory: Education in a Lean State*, Aurora, Ontario: Garamond Press.

Tomlinson, S. (2004) Comprehensive success: bog-standard government, in M. Benn and C. Chitty (eds) *A Tribute to Caroline Benn: Education and Democracy*, London: Continuum.

Tymms, P. (2004) Are standards rising in English primary schools? *British Educational Research Journal*, 30 (4): 477–94.

Vygotsky, L. (1978) *Mind in Society: The Development of Higher Psychological Processes*, M. Cole, V. John-Steiner, S. Scribner and E. Souberman (eds and trans.), Cambridge MA: Harvard University Press.

—— (1986) *Thought and Language*, A. Kozulin (ed. and trans.), Cambridge MA: Massachusetts Institute of Technology Press.

Wrigley, T. (2003) *Schools of Hope: A New Agenda for School Improvement*, Stoke-on-Trent: Trentham.

4.3   The rights of the child

Rightfully mine!

Heather Montgomery

The idea that children are bearers of rights rather than objects of concern is relatively recent but it is one that has been enormously influential. In terms of national and international policy, children's rights are central to discussions of how to improve children's lives and, within academia, the idea that children are passive subjects to be analysed and discussed has been firmly rejected. Implementation of these rights however is far from straightforward and there has been much debate over exactly which rights children have and whether or not it is possible to set worldwide standards for all children or to talk meaningfully about universal rights. This chapter will discuss some of these issues in relation to the United Nations Convention on the Rights of the Child (abbreviated to the UNCRC or the Convention). This is, of course, one piece of legislation among many and all countries have their own national rights but the UNCRC is the inspiration behind these national laws and is the most significant, and controversial, piece of international children's rights legislation.

Children's rights and human rights

In the aftermath of the Second World War the idea that everyone had legal, inalienable rights as a result of their humanity was codified in international law. Although the notion of rights was not new and it is possible to talk about human rights in Ancient Greece, or as a fundamental underpinning to the French or American Revolutions, after the horrors of the war there was a desire to codify the principle that all people, by virtue of their humanity, had certain inalienable rights, such as the right to life or the right to freedom of conscience. These rights depended not on the property they owned, the colour of their skin, or their sex but on the simple fact that they were human. Guided by this vision the General Assembly of the United Nations adopted the Universal Declaration of Human Rights on 10 December 1948. The Declaration was guided by four main principles: that rights are universal (they apply equally to everyone); inalienable (they cannot be taken away arbitrarily); indivisible (governments cannot pick and choose which rights they enforce); and interdependent (supplementary rights cannot conflict with the universal principles of human rights law).

A complex web of international legislation has grown up since the 1948 Declaration and there are now various international treaties and conventions which focus on rights for specific groups. The Geneva Convention Relative to the Treatment of Prisoners of War (1951), the Refugee Convention (1951) and the UNCRC (1989) are among the most famous. This chapter will focus on the last of these, which is now an integral part of the human rights discourse, as well as a culmination of six decades of work for children's rights and special protection for children. It was opened for signature in 1979 and has been signed and ratified (incorporated into national law) by every country in the world except the USA and Somalia. Since its adoption in 1989 there have been supplementary conventions and protocols adopted which include special provision for especially vulnerable children, such as the 2000 Optional Protocols to the Convention which increased protection available to children involved in armed conflicts and at risk of sexual exploitation.

The UNCRC states that all children have the same rights as adults and in addition that the child has distinct rights 'by reason of his physical and mental immaturity, [and] needs special safeguards and care, including appropriate legal protection' (Preamble). The Convention is made up of 54 legally binding articles covering, among other things, children's right to healthcare, education, nationality and legal representation but the fundamental principle behind the Convention is stated in Article 3, which reads 'All actions concerning the child shall take full account of his or her best interests', meaning that adults who act on behalf of children should always act in ways that place the child's welfare and best interests above all other considerations. The rights set out in the UNCRC are often grouped into four categories known as the '4 Ps' of children's rights: their right to *provision* (i.e. their rights to food, housing or education); their right to *protection* (against exploitation and abuse); their right to *prevention* (the systems that must be put in place to prevent abuse or infringements of their rights such as a right to legal representation or privacy); and (the most controversial) their right to *participation* (the right of children to take part in decisions made on their behalf) (Burr and Montgomery 2003).

Activity 4.3.1: The UNCRC

The UNCRC is a much discussed and invoked document and it is worth reading in full in order to understand its provisions. It is equally important to look at what it does not claim for children. You can find a copy of the document at various United Nations websites, including that of the Office of the United Nations High Commissioner for Human Rights (http://www.unhchr.ch/html/menu3/b/k2crc.htm) or see the photo-essay available at the UNICEF website (http://www.unicef.org/crc/).

The Convention is in two parts; the first sets out the rights that children have and the second discusses how these rights will be measured and monitored. Read through the Convention and as you do so think about whether you notice any gaps in it or anything that you think should be there but is not. Why do you think, for example, that love and happiness are mentioned in the Preamble but nowhere else in the Convention?

Comment

The UNCRC is an official document that sets out legally enforceable standards. It is important to distinguish this set of legal standards with the sometimes loose way that the phrase children's rights is used, to refer, for instance, to children's right to a happy home or to loving parents. There is an important difference between rights and wants and it is essential to differentiate between the desire for children's well-being and the legal responsibility to enforce this. It is possible to say, for example, that a child has a right to an adequate standard of living but it is not meaningful to say a child has a right to a happy childhood, no matter how desirable this might be. As Jack Donnelly argues:

We do not have human rights to all things that are good, or even all *important* good things.

For example, we are not entitled – do not have (human) rights – to love, charity or compassion. Parents who abuse the trust of children wreak havoc with millions of lives every day. We do not, however, have a human right to loving, supportive parents. In fact, to recognize such a right would transform family relations in ways that many people would find unappealing or even destructive.

(2003: 10–11)

When drafting the Convention its authors were very careful therefore not to set up a right to something that is legally meaningless. The Preamble states an ideal and recognizes that in a perfect world all children would grow up in 'an atmosphere of happiness, love and understanding' but this is not, and never can be, a legally enforceable standard.

Problems and pitfalls

The UNCRC has been so successful because its basic premise seems uncontroversial. It is hard to argue that children should not be entitled to special protective measures, that they do not have a right to food, shelter or education. Yet, despite the fact that it is the most signed and ratified piece of human rights legislation in history, implementation has not always been easy. As the activity above suggested, rights are different from something that is simply desirable, or even morally correct. Rights are entitlements and cannot be understood without reference to responsibility. If one person has a right to something then someone, or some other body, has a duty to ensure that right. In ratifying the UNCRC national governments are not simply saying that they support children's rights in theory – they are agreeing to change national laws and to devote the necessary resources to promoting and enforcing these rights. Their attempts to do so are scrutinized every five years by the United Nations Committee on the Rights of the Child who have found that, despite the rhetoric, many governments have failed to fulfil their obligations, sometimes through practical factors such as a lack of resources and sometimes because they have lodged reservations to certain aspects of the Convention.

Although children's rights legislation, like all human rights legislation, claims to be universal and indivisible, ensuring that governments cannot pick and choose which rights they enforce and which they do not, in practice, and in order to get as many countries as possible to sign up for the legislation, states are allowed to lodge reservations. This means that states can effectively opt out of ratifying certain articles which conflict with their cultural beliefs or their national law. The majority of countries have entered reservations against particular aspects of the UNCRC so that, for instance, Saudi Arabia lodged a blanket reservation against any articles that it views as incompatible with the requirements of Islamic Sharia law. The UK also initially lodged reservations about the detention of young people alongside adults, claiming that it had inadequate resources to ensure this segregation. Since criticism from the United Nations Committee on the Rights of the Child in 2002, however, the UK government has made great efforts to ensure that children and adults are not locked up together and in 2007 argued that this reservation was no longer needed.

Reservations, such as those lodged by Saudi Arabia, touch on an aspect of the UNCRC which has been criticized by academics and activists outside the West who have claimed that the Convention is based on the liberal, humanist values of the West which have limited meaning in societies where there are very different understandings of the relationships between parents and children and between people and the state. Erica Burman (1996) has argued that the UNCRC is based on the notion that each human is an individual who has the right to liberty, to shelter and to freedom of expression, yet this understanding of the person as an autonomous individual does not easily translate into other societies (see also Boyden 1997). In many countries the child is not seen as a self-sufficient individual with rights independent of the family but is viewed as being embedded in a web of relationships, which come with duties, obligations, and sometimes the expectation of sacrifice on behalf of the family. In his work on the UNCRC in Japan, anthropologist Roger Goodman has commented that:

> ... when the concept of 'rights' was introduced into Japan ... a whole new vocabulary had to be developed to explain it, as did the idea of the individual who could be endowed with such rights. Even today, individualism has strongly negative connections in Japan and is frequently associated with western concepts of selfishness.
>
> (1996: 131)

Others have gone further and argued that the UNCRC is part of the power struggle between the industrialized countries of the North (the minority world) and those of the South (the majority world) in which the values of the former are foisted onto the latter in a new form of neo-colonialism (Pupavac 2001). Rebecca Wallace sums up this debate:

> The countries of the South contend that the wealthy countries of North adopt the moral high ground and use human rights instruments as sticks with which to beat them. The North is accused of low intensity political warfare in which the South is cast as the villain, while the North's image is that of a paragon of morality and enlightenment, a successful Euro-American civilisation, which has got all the 'fundamentals right'.
>
> (2001: 11)

Western countries stand accused of interfering in the private relationships of families in the majority world and imposing on them definitions of childhood that are very different from locally understood concepts. In doing so, as Judith Ennew notes; 'Childhood becomes a valuable commodity in the power structures of relationships between developed and developing countries' (1986: 23). Opposition to the Convention is not restricted only to the countries of the South, however, but has also come from the USA which, although it signed the Convention in 1995, has refused to ratify it on the grounds that it violates principles of national sovereignty and the rights of individual states. It further claims that children's rights are best protected within families, by parents, not by the state.

Given all of the above it is not surprising that the most controversial right discussed in the Convention concerns participation. Although the UNCRC does not define participation explicitly, Article 12 states: 'The child has the right to express his or her opinion freely and to have that opinion taken into account in any matter or procedure affecting the child.' Other articles also affirm a young person's right to freedom of expression (Article 13), to freedom of association (Article 15) and to access appropriate information (Article 17). Such rights have proved most difficult to implement because issues such as the ideal relationship between people, particularly between adults and children, remain contested, as do the expectations on children and the conceptualizations of childhood. Looking at non-Western societies there are many instances where children are not seen as individuals in their own right, where they are not seen as having any right to be consulted in matters concerning them and where they are viewed as their parents' dependants, and sometimes even their property (Montgomery 2008). Within Western societies also ideas about the extent to which children should be consulted and listened to remain problematic (see the case study at the end of the chapter) and there is still a reluctance to view children as equal participants in society. There can be a tension between rights of participation and protection and there may be instances where, regardless of young people's right to express an opinion, this right is superseded in what adults perceive are their best interests. In Norway, for instance, the Children's Ombudsman pushed for a legal ban on cosmetic surgery for those under 18 despite protests from girls of 16 who felt fully competent to make informed decisions about their bodies (Montgomery 2003).

It can be argued that the UNCRC presents an idealized vision rather than a blueprint of practical policy and those who drafted it were well aware of the problems discussed above. The concept of 'evolving capacities' mentioned in Article 5 has now become part of the children's rights agenda with both academics and activists beginning to look at how this can help the implementation and understanding of children's rights (Lansdown 2005). The UNCRC recognizes that children at different ages have different capacities, especially in the extent to which they can be consulted about decisions which affect them. This depends not only on their physical and emotional development but also on cultural expectations. Children in the majority world are often expected to work for the family and carry out skilful tasks, such as the care of younger siblings, or cooking food, at much younger ages than their peers in the West and the concept of evolving capacities goes some way towards dealing with problems of local realities and cultural differences.

What is a child?

The heterogeneous nature of childhood and the vast difference in capacities and capabilities between a baby and an 18-year-old have also proved problematic in implementing a convention that applies equally to all children. The UNCRC defines childhood as follows: 'A child is recognized as a person under 18, unless national laws recognize the age of majority earlier.' In bureaucratic terms this is a neat division and it supports the fundamental philosophy of the UNCRC that concepts such as children's rights are not negotiable at local level. However, it does not allow for issues of cultural difference which, as the discussion above suggested, have led to criticisms that the boundaries of childhood have been fixed externally and the parameters of a 'normal' childhood have been set by outsiders with limited understandings of local cultural norms. The idea that a person aged 17 is a child is ludicrous in many cultures where that 'child' may have been married for several years, be a mother or father, or an economically productive worker.

While many have challenged the idea of a fixed boundary to mark the end of childhood, an equally important, although much less studied, issue is the question of when childhood begins. For many reasons, not least personal politics, the question of the start of childhood is, on the whole, one that those who work on children's rights have avoided. The UNCRC is vague on the subject. The Preamble states that 'the child needs special safeguards and care, including appropriate legal protection, before as well as after birth' but it does not enshrine this as a legal right in the Convention as it would be unacceptable to those states that allow abortion. Indeed on signing the Convention the UK explicitly stated that it 'interprets the Convention as applicable only following a live birth'. The UK government thus takes the position that childhood starts at birth and only at this point

154   H. Montgomery

does a child have full legal protection and rights. This legal definition is a problematic one however and has been deeply contested. There are those who recognize a foetus as fully human from the moment of conception (the position of the modern Catholic Church) while others see the foetus as developing into a child more gradually. The 2008 debates in the UK over abortion and whether or not to lower the legal limits of abortion from 24 to 20 weeks centred around the issue of when a foetus became a person and when, and if, the state should give full legal protection to the unborn. Members of Parliament rejected the lowering of the legal abortion limit but the exact status of a foetus between 24 and 40 weeks gestation remains ambiguous; it has some protection in law but it is not a legally recognized child with rights.

Such a discussion might seem well off the subject of the UNCRC but it shows very clearly that the very notion of childhood is contested, as are the exact rights to which children are entitled, depending on their age and stage in life. These issues are also extremely pertinent to the case study I will now discuss, based on work carried out by Priscilla Alderson, Joanna Hawthorn and Margaret Killen, in which they worked with neonatal and premature babies and examined the controversial question of whether premature babies are citizens with rights, including those of participation. The researchers based their study on ethnographic work in four neonatal intensive care units (NICUs) during 2002–4, looking at babies who were born prematurely. They examined how these babies were conceptualized by those looking after them and the impact this had on the care they were given. They also analysed whether these children's rights were being respected and implemented and how such young babies could usefully be brought into discussions of agency and citizenship.

On the face of it such issues may seem irrelevant or even absurd. Few would deny that a baby, once born, should be given every help to survive and indeed the right to life is an absolute in all human rights legislation. Yet the question is not that simple and, as the authors point out, 'Premature babies, born as early as 22 or 23 weeks gestation, are the same gestational age as the fetus that has no rights' (Alderson, et al. 2005a: 71). Furthermore they argue that the right to life is not absolute for the prematurely born. Article 6 of the UNCRC states that 'every child has the inherent right to life [and] to the maximum extent possible survival and development' but this is not always achievable. The authors discuss the policies in several neonatal units about whether or not to treat those children born at 23 or 24 weeks and whether their right to life is over-ridden by the question of their best interests and long-term futures. The authors point to the potential conflicts between the provisions in the UNCRC for survival and those which ensure quality of life, such as Article 6 which talks about the best possible development of the child, Article 24 which deals with the highest standards of healthcare and Article 27 which claims an adequate standard of living for all children. Medical personnel and parents must decide, when dealing with such premature babies, about whether or not to intervene or to withdraw any treatment given so far. This can range from allowing the baby to die by removing artificial ventilation to withholding fluids and nutrition thereby actively hastening the child's death.

Alderson, et al. then go on to discuss other ways in which children's rights are not always seen as being applicable to the newly born. They discuss how being socially marginalized or from certain ethnic minorities increases a child's chance of being born prematurely. Although there is no discrimination within the NICUs and all children are treated equally, the chances of them being there at all are heavily dependent on external factors and on poverty and unequal social relationships outside the unit, implying that

the UNCRC's articles on non-discrimination and equality are not being fully implemented. Between NICUs there are also differences so that some neonatal units do their
best to ensure close and supportive relationships between parents and children, such as
encouraging mothers to breastfeed their children, while others do not. In some cases the
lighting is very bright, or the unit noisy and the babies seem to show signs of distress at
this, while at others, the atmosphere is calmer. As the authors conclude:

> Staff in bright noisy units tend to dismiss research evidence about the discomfort
> to the babies, and to discuss the need to attract and retain staff by making the units
> friendly cheerful places for them to work in. This is an important argument, adequate
> staffing levels are vital for the welfare of the babies and staff, but it appears to assume
> that the babies' need and possibly right to a quiet dim environment conflicts with
> and is less important than reasonable working conditions for the staff.
>
> (2005a: 77)

So far, this argument is not particularly controversial – ensuring the highest standards
for premature babies and deciding treatment based on their best interests is exactly in
line with what is demanded by the UNCRC. What makes Alderson, *et al.*'s work more
problematic is their insistence on looking beyond premature babies' basic care needs and
focusing on the wider rights of all children to be seen as citizens and to participate in
decisions made about them. The authors are not arguing that premature babies can make
informed decisions over their treatment or even that they are aware of what is going on
around them but they do argue for a rethinking of what children's rights to participation might mean in this context. They argue that babies can communicate and make, on
some level, a decision about their treatment and that far from being passive recipients
of care, they seem to express particular likes and dislikes. One baby, for example, did
not like his feet being touched, another one responded differently to different doctors
and nurses and seemingly expressed a preference for one nurse over others. The authors
claim that both parents and paediatricians see these babies as independent, autonomous
beings who appear to fight and cling to life against sometimes overwhelming odds. 'Many
parents and practitioners … gave examples of babies continuing to survive against all
expectations, or sometimes unexpectedly "giving up" as if, in some ways, the babies had
the final say in whether they lived or died' (2005b: 39). One mother said of her son's
determination to live:

> 'Yes, I think he definitely chose to live, because there were a couple of points where
> I would have exited. I have to say I would have left this life …. He was incredibly
> ill … he was dying effectively, and the doctors were saying that, "You know it's not
> good," and I kind of got this feeling that he had decided, "No actually I am not ready
> to go. I want to live," because then he would come back in from his sort of dying,
> and he would be fine. Well not quite but he would be different, and I feel that he
> chose to live … he's just incredibly determined.'
>
> (2005b: 45)

These babies are obviously limited in terms of the ways they can communicate and participate and it may be meaningless to talk about citizenship, participation or children's
rights in this context. Alderson, *et al.* are very aware of the problems inherent in their
argument and write that 'Rights language can irritate and alienate its opponents who

dismiss claims that children have rights as empty slogans in search of a meaning. Rights and citizenship, especially of older children, may be denigrated and trivialised if applied to babies' (2005a: 79). What their work shows very clearly however is that if rights are to be taken seriously for all children, then no one group of children can be excluded, even the very young. Premature babies are often seen as being an anomalous group for whom the absolute right to life is, in fact, negotiable and which their carers may revoke. By viewing them as bearers of rights, and possibly even as citizens, there is an acknowledgement that they are agents who influence their own lives as well as those around them. Alderson, *et al.* make no overblown claims that premature babies need to be consulted over their treatment or demand rights for them which do not exist and they cannot benefit from but they do argue for an acknowledgement of these babies' personhood, individuality and abilities. They conclude:

> … part of being a rights-holder is to have some say in how one's rights are defined and respected. There is a transfer of some acknowledged expertise and authority to the child. The neonatal examples suggest that babies too can have unique insight into their best interests, and adults need to take account of these if their decisions about care are to be adequately informed and humane. Informed neonatal care is then an interdependent partnership, with the adults referring to the baby's contributions.
>
> Needs and interests may be arbitrary, rights are principled and formally agreed entitlements and standards, as in the UNCRC.
>
> Rights further involve respect and dignity as well as care, when babies are perceived as rights holders, and to some extent as persons and citizens. The recognition entails listening seriously to baby's expressions of pain or pleasure and responding appropriately.
>
> (2005a: 79)

Conclusion

This chapter has argued that children's rights, while generally acknowledged as a positive force for improving children's lives, are not straightforward to implement and remain contested at an ideological level. Conceptualizing children as active participants remains especially problematic and by using the admittedly extreme case study of premature babies I have argued that not only are there problems with cross-cultural and universal understandings of rights but that within societies there is also ideological and practical resistance to the idea that all children are rights bearers. The example of premature babies may be extreme but it is useful in that it shows that supporting children's rights is not simply about providing basic services or attending to their needs or welfare. Instead it is about re-conceptualizing notions of childhood, viewing children as equals to adults and recognizing their agency and views, however they are expressed. Such a rethink would be far-reaching and goes against long-standing beliefs both in the UK and abroad but the UNCRC, for all its problems, is a radical document which calls on adults not to 'give' rights to children but to empower them to take up their place as equal members of society.

Student reflection

• Why do you think there is opposition to children having rights?

Key points

• The UNCRC states that all children have the same rights as adults, in addition to specific rights known as the 4 Ps: provision, protection, prevention and participation.

• The right to entitlement cannot be understood without responsibility and despite an almost universal signing of the UNCRC many governments have failed to fulfil their obligations.

• In many countries the child is not seen as an independent individual with rights within the family. The USA claims that children's rights are best protected by parents and not the state.

• Issues surround the definition of children's rights, especially that of participation, with tension between the rights of the child to be heard and the rights of the child to be protected.

• It can be argued that the UNCRC presents an idealized vision rather than a blueprint of practical policy although it recognizes that children of different ages have different capabilities.

• In the majority of cases, childhood refers to those under 18, however the idea of a fixed boundary is problematic for both the start and end of childhood.

• There is tension around the rights of very premature babies and this helps to illustrate the differing views of the right for a child to be 'listened to' in addition to be cared for.

Recommended reading

Alderson, P. (2008) *Young Children's Rights: Exploring Beliefs, Principles and Practice*, 2nd edn, London: Jessica Kingsley Publishers.

Montgomery, H. (2001) 'Imposing rights? A case study of child prostitution in Thailand', in J. Cowan, M.-B. Dembour, and R. Wilson (eds) *Culture and Rights*, Cambridge: Cambridge University Press.

Pupavac, V. (2001) 'Misanthropy without borders: the international children's rights regime', *Disasters*, 25 (2): 95–112.

Woodhead, M. (1997) 'Psychology and the cultural construction of children's needs', in A. James and A. Prout (eds) *Constructing and Deconstructing Childhood: Contemporary Issues in the Sociological Study of Childhood*, London: Falmer Press.

References

Alderson, P., Hawthorne, J. and Killen, M. (2005a) 'Are premature babies citizens with rights? Provision rights and the edges of citizenship', *Journal of Social Sciences*, 9: 71–81.

—— (2005b) 'The participation rights of premature babies', *The International Journal of Children's Rights*, 13: 31–50.

Boyden, J. (1997) 'Childhood and the policy makers: a comparative perspective on the globalization of childhood', in A. James and A. Prout (eds) *Constructing and Deconstructing Childhood: Contemporary Issues in the Sociological Study of Childhood*, London: Falmer Press.

Burman, E. (1996) 'Local, global and globalized: child development and international child rights legislation', *Childhood*, 3: 45–66.

Burr, R. and Montgomery, H. (2003) 'Children and rights', in M. Woodhead and H. Montgomery (eds) *Understanding Childhood: An Interdisciplinary Approach*, Chichester: John Wiley.

Donnelly, J. (2003) *Universal Human Rights in Theory and Practice*, 2nd edn, Ithaca: Cornell University Press.

Ennew, J. (1986) *Sexual Exploitation of Children*, Cambridge: Polity Press.

Goodman, R. (1996) 'On introducing the UN Convention on the Rights of the Child into Japan', in R. Goodman and I. Neary (eds) *Case Studies on Human Rights in Japan*, Richmond: Japan Library, Curzon Press.

Lansdown, G. (2005) *The Evolving Capacities of the Child*, Florence: UNICEF Innocenti Research Centre.

Montgomery, H. (2003) 'Intervening in children's lives', in H. Montgomery, R. Burr and M. Woodhead (eds) *Changing Childhoods: Global and Local*, Chichester: John Wiley.

—— (2008) *An Introduction to Childhood: Anthropological Perspectives on Children's Lives*, Oxford: Blackwell.

Pupavac, V. (2001) 'Misanthropy without borders: the international children's rights regime', *Disasters*, 25 (2): 95–112.

UN Convention on the Rights of the Child (UNCRC) (1990) Convention on the Rights of the Child. Available online at: http://www2.ohchr.org/english/law/crc.htm (accessed 18.09.2009).

Wallace, R. (2001) 'Human rights and responsibilities: the inextricable link', *Human Rights and UK Practice*, 2 (3): 9–12.

4.4 Childhood and youth poverty in the UK

The have nots

Diane Grant

Background

Around the turn of the nineteenth century little state provision existed to provide a 'safety net' for the poor. At that time children were expected to help towards the family budget, often working long hours in extremely dangerous jobs and in difficult situations for a meagre wage. It was left to charitable organizations to try and plug the gaps. The Waifs and Strays Society was one of the first charitable organizations established to try to alleviate child poverty on a national scale. They highlighted the plight of the climbing boys who were employed to sweep chimneys, and that of the children in the mills who crawled under the heavy machinery (while in motion), to retrieve cotton bobbins. Both boys and girls were employed in the coal mines, scrambling their way through tunnels which were too narrow and low for adults. Children were often required to work to supplement the family income by doing ad hoc work such as flower or match selling or shoe shining (Hidden Lives).

The organization is now known as the Children's Society and is one of 120 organizations that signed up to a declaration to end child poverty. It continues to work with the most disadvantaged and poor children in society, noting in its February 2008 report on destitution among asylum-seeking and refugee children that:

> Children were frequently hungry. Some children were only able to eat once a day and sometimes their parents did not eat for several days on end. Children did not have the space, resources or opportunities to play and develop. Some children did not have access to healthcare or education, and were not able to learn English or to read and write in any language.
>
> (The Children's Society 2008)

Activity 4.4.1: Child poverty in the UK

- How would you define child poverty in current UK society?
- How does child poverty manifest itself?
- What do you think are the consequences of child poverty?

Child poverty today is in many ways different from poverty at the turn of the twentieth century, in that it is not acceptable for children to work and there are rules and regulations which govern their well-being. Yet, in a country which is rated as one of the strongest EU economies and one of the richest countries in the world there now exists great inequality of opportunity which prevents young people in the UK from ever achieving their potential – unless there is change.

Historically, debates on poverty have centred on the victim-blaming ethos initially encountered by Rowntree in 1899, in which policy makers strenuously believed that poverty existed because people mismanaged and wasted their incomes on non-necessities. They had steadfastly refused to acknowledge the existence of poverty on any terms, believing simply to determine the phenomenon as being caused solely by the fecklessness of the poor. Rowntree had begun his quest for the definitive explanation of primary (absolute) poverty in 1899, yet in his following two surveys he began to include some elements of social need rather than just measuring the needs for physical efficiency – the needs of food, fuel, clothing, rent and household sundries. Following Rowntree's final study in 1951 he found that poverty had drastically declined. This was due in great part to full employment, the implementation of state welfare and improvements in housing and health. Since his work, poverty studies have used a variety of measures with which to determine the extent of poverty in the UK (Rowntree 1901; 1937; Rountree and Lavers 1951).

In the 1960s Abel-Smith and Townsend devised a poverty line based upon an income level below 140 per cent of supplementary benefit rates; in the 1970s Townsend developed a Deprivation Index, which was based upon cultural norms, and in the 1980s Mack and Lansley adopted a consensual measurement based upon opinions of the public. In all of these measurements the need for both physical as well as social nourishment was recognized. The poverty and social exclusion survey carried out by the Joseph Rowntree Foundation in 1999 used a method to define and measure poverty based on socially perceived necessities, which allowed for the definition of childhood poverty to be democratically decided by the design of a poverty line specifically related to the needs of children rather than adults or households. The meaning of poverty in children's lives could therefore be better understood (Gordon, *et al.* 2000).

According to Alcock (1993), commentators do not always agree that poverty exists in modern Britain and this influences the way they wish to address it or not (ibid.: 1). The evidence of improving living standards over the twentieth century is dramatic, and incontrovertible. When the pressure groups say that one-third of the population is living in poverty, they cannot be saying that one-third of people are living below the draconian subsistence levels used by Booth and Rowntree (Moore 1989: 5, cited in Alcock 1993: 3).

Moore's argument was that the problem of poverty was, and continued to be, dealt with through welfare policy and through the social security system, therefore no further action was needed. Yet poverty persisted and academics such as Veit-Wilson (1998) argued that 'any government claiming to want to act against it must set out minimum income standards to identify the problems, guide the solutions and monitor the effects'. However poverty campaigners in the 1990s found great difficulty in obtaining evidence on how minimum needs were calculated and incorporated within welfare benefits. It was left to committed campaigners such as Suzi Leather (member of the Consumer Panel of the Ministry of Agriculture, Fisheries and Food) to try pin down the government on how much they estimated a family could spend on food when living on benefits and Boardman (1992) to highlight the impact of fuel poverty on poor households (Leather 1992; Boardman 1992).

Among the public in Britain today there is scepticism about the existence of poverty, although relatively unacknowledged. The assumptions are that people are poor because they are somehow inferior, thus discrimination in the form of 'povertyism' emerges and affects the lives of people in a similar way to racism, sexism or ageism, denying people rights and opportunities and thus creating social exclusion (Stitt and Grant 1993; Lister 2008; Hennessy and Grant 2006; Sayer 2005).

Social exclusion is experienced by children in all aspects of their lives, for instance school, and in the wider community. According to Ridge (2002) the lack of money makes it difficult to take part in and enjoy activities with friends or to maintain and sustain friendships; poverty thus makes it difficult to behave in normal childhood ways. The desire to shield children from discrimination and the stigma attached to being poor thus results in measures by parents to try and ameliorate 'visible' poverty. This often attracts criticism from those not willing to acknowledge the existence of poverty, who then condemn any consumption of non-basic goods as unnecessary, thus validating their beliefs.

Poverty campaigners throughout history have endeavoured to define what poverty is and determine how many people fall below what is commonly known as the poverty 'line'. Peter Townsend's major contribution to the poverty debate emerged in Margaret Thatcher's first term of office with a new Conservative government. He argued that poverty was not simply a lack of money to purchase basic needs, as Rowntree had defined in his primary poverty measure, but was the lack of resources with which to participate in social activities deemed normal in modern society. Although both of these scholarly publications have enhanced and illuminated the academic debate on the many privations of poverty, using a variety of measurements, at the time neither were policy-specific. However Townsend's definition was later used to form the foundation of a relative measure which was developed by Mack and Lansley (1985) and more recently by Gordon, *et al.* (2000), thus Townsend's contribution now forms the basis of a measurement used by government to determine the numbers of children experiencing material deprivation in Britain (DWP 2008; CPAG 2008).

Much campaigning on behalf of children has been undertaken, most notably by the Child Poverty Action Group (CPAG) and the Joseph Rowntree Foundation (JRF). There were major achievements throughout the twentieth century, including the political impetus to improve the welfare of all citizens through the implementation of the National Health Service, Social Services, improvements in housing conditions and in access to education (Thane 1982).

When Labour swept to power in 1997 they had inherited a situation in which child poverty in the UK had tripled between 1979 and 1995 (Bradbury and Jäntti 1999). One in every five children in the UK were living in a workless household and one in three children were living in relative poverty. The UK had the highest teenage pregnancy rate across Europe (Social Exclusion Unit 1999). The political *will* to change the fortunes of such children became clear when in 1999 the then Prime Minister Tony Blair made a pledge that his government would eradicate child poverty in this generation. He committed the government to breaking 'the cycle of deprivation so that children born into poverty are not condemned to social exclusion and deprivation' (Tony Blair 1999).

The government had set about developing a National Childcare Strategy in 1998 with the remit to expand choices for parents and improve the prospects of children through raising the quality of childcare, making it more affordable and more accessible. Labour's initial reforms adopted 'joined up' approaches to services, which would ensure government departments would work with each other and with both the private and voluntary sectors. One of the first steps was to enable the Department for Work and Pensions and Her Majesty's Treasury to share a Public Service Agreement (PSA) aimed at reducing the number of children in low-income households by at least a quarter by 2004–5 and to halve it by 2010 (Magadi and Middleton 2007).

> The Government's view is that the chief cause of child poverty is worklessness. There is strong evidence to support this, but other causes are also apparent. Since … even the most affluent people may be workless, it is necessary to look more broadly at other causes which often interact with worklessness, such as marital and relationship breakdown, unstable parenting, inadequate levels of educational attainment and healthcare provision, and involvement in crime.
>
> (House of Commons Work and Pensions Select Committee 2004: 20)

In 2004 the Chancellor Gordon Brown re-iterated his party's commitment by spelling out the disadvantages heaped on poor children when he gave the Joseph Rowntree Lecture entitled 'Our children are our future' on 8 July:

> … an infant who grows up in a poor family is less likely to stay on at school, or even attend school regularly, less likely to get qualifications and go to college, more likely to be trapped in the worst job or no job at all, more likely to be trapped in a cycle of deprivation that is life long … less likely to reach his or her full potential, a young child's chances crippled even before their life's journey has barely begun …

At the 2008 Labour Party Conference, after having succeeded Tony Blair as Prime Minister in 2007, Gordon Brown qualified his commitment to eliminating child poverty:

> For me, the fairer future starts with putting children first – with the biggest investment in children this country has ever seen. It means delivering the best possible starts in life with services tailored to the needs of every single precious child.

Thus the main thrust of New Labour's anti-poverty strategy has been to address child poverty, with the weight of evidence highlighting how being socially excluded in childhood perversely affects the life chances and opportunities of future generations. The government's child poverty strategy is mainly focused on children in families aged 0–15, while poverty among young people aged 16–25 continues to receive relatively limited attention. Recent policy interventions designed to tackle the multiple facets of social exclusion have resulted in a raft of policy measures set out into four main themes:

- support for parents to participate in the labour market
- provision of financial support
- improved public services, whose aims are to improve life chances for children
- provision of support for parents in parenting skills development.

All of these are designed to support the effort to eradicate child poverty.

Much of the academic literature relating to child poverty has focused on two issues: the identification of households where risk is greatest and research into the so-called 'scarring' of children and the transmission of disadvantage into adulthood.

Identification of households at risk of poverty is now well established (Lloyd 2006; Bradshaw 2006; Platt 2007; Iavacou and Berthoud 2006). By 1998 over one-third of children in Britain were living within households whose incomes fell below 50 per cent of the average income, the measure then most commonly used. The measurement of poverty in 2008 was measured against three indicators:

- When children live in households with 'needs adjusted' incomes whose incomes fall below 60 per cent of the current national median income. These are described as children experiencing *relative low income*.
- When income falls below 70 per cent of the national median income and where children are experiencing material deprivation and relative low income.[1]
- When children are in households with a 'needs adjusted' income below 60 per cent of the 1998–9 national median income increased for price inflation.

(CPAG 2008)

To determine whether material deprivation exists in the household, families who have income of under 70 per cent of the current national median are asked what they do not have from a list of 21 items (see Table 4.4.1). The items a family does not have are given a weighting and scored and this enables a count of materially deprived children.

While the impetus to eradicate child poverty is welcomed, the measures have had some criticism in that they do not take into account housing costs and therefore do not show the real disposable income of households (CPAG 2008). In the UK, 22 per cent of children live in poverty, however rates vary across the UK with London and the North West and North East of England and Wales having child poverty rates of 25 per cent and above (DWP 2008). If the measurement advocated by the CPAG were used, which includes housing costs, then these figures rise to 41 per cent for London, 48 per cent for inner London and 29 per cent to 38 per cent for the remaining areas identified.

Not only is location a factor in poverty, so too is household composition and characteristics. Households where there are three or more children, or children under five and parents who are in receipt of benefits or disabled have higher proportions of children in poverty. Similarly, whether the child's household is Bangladeshi or Pakistani or Black (non-Caribbean) is also a factor. Other demographic data highlights inequalities, for example where a child resides in an owner-occupied house, 14 per cent of children are known to have a relatively low income family compared to a staggering 51 per cent of children being at risk of poverty who live in rented accommodation from the local authority (CPAG 2008).

The 'scarring' effect of child poverty shows that the manifestation of financial inequality, and the material deprivation it creates, inhibits both child development and educational attainment. Educational attainment is lower for poorer children; they have fewer opportunities, with child poverty heralded as a root cause of disadvantage in later life and a result of the social exclusion of the parent(s), low parental income and job instability.

Finally, in addition to child poverty, concerns have been raised as to the numbers of youths experiencing poverty as well as the increased proportion of young people leaving school without adequate training or qualifications. The latter group have been referred to as NEET, short for 'not in education, employment or training'. The first government statistics for young people who are NEET were released on 19 June 2008 and show that around 10 per cent of young people fell into this category, which accounts for around 189,500 young people (DCSF 2008). Being poor in the transition years between childhood and adulthood can have serious consequences and some argue the ways in which the government deals with youth poverty emphasize a disconnection from mainstream society does not address the key issue of income deprivation.

Table 4.4.1 Proportion of children whose parents report they do not have and cannot afford items

		Poorest fifth	2nd	3rd	4th	Richest fifth	All children
Child-level	Outdoor space/facilities to play	25	17	12	8	4	15
	Enough bedrooms for every child 10 years or over and of a different gender	28	17	9	2	3	15
	Celebrations on special occasions	9	4	2	1	0	4
	Leisure equipment such as sports equipment or a bicycle	15	7	2	1	0	6
	At least one week's holiday away from home with family	55	41	22	11	4	32
	Hobby or leisure activity	14	6	2	1	1	6
	Swimming at least once a month	21	12	5	1	1	10
	Have friends round for tea or a snack once a fortnight	15	8	3	1	0	7
	Go on a school trip at least once a term	14	6	3	1	0	6
	Go to a playgroup at least once a week	11	7	3	1	0	6
Parental-level	Money to decorate home	35	21	13	6	2	18
	Hobby or leisure activity	31	22	12	5	3	17
	Holiday away from home one week a year not with relatives	64	48	29	16	6	38
	Home contents insurance	42	20	7	3	0	18
	Friends round for a drink/meal at least once a month	29	18	9	5	1	15
	Make savings of £10 a month or more	66	50	29	16	8	40

(continued)

	Poorest fifth	2nd	3rd	4th	Richest fifth	All children
Parental-level Two pairs of all-weather shoes for each adult	19	11	4	1	1	9
Replace worn-out furniture	51	35	21	13	5	30
Replace broken electrical goods	42	26	13	6	3	22
Money to spend on self each week	56	41	23	11	4	32
Keep house warm	17	8	3	2	1	8

Source: Department for Work and Pensions, Households Below Average Income: an analysis of the income distribution 1994/95–2006/07, National Statistics, 2008.

Economic disadvantage

There are some limitations when using household income to measure poverty among children. Initially it assumes that children will share the same living standards of their family – if the family or household is poor, it naturally follows that children in that household must also be poor. In other words, it is assumed that household income is distributed evenly among household members. Yet there is evidence to suggest that spending on children is relatively similar across all families. Further evidence highlights how women's share of family income is disproportionately small (Stitt and Grant 1993; Grant and Maxwell 1998; Goode, *et al.* 1998; Middleton, *et al.* 1997).

> 'There are times when I've said to him [husband] that I don't feel like a tea, and he sees that I've given them [children] all the tea. He'll say, "where's your tea?" and I'll have a piece of toast … that causes more trouble then. He feels guilty he says I'm starving myself, I say, "I'm not, I'm eating toast aren't I?".'
> (Couple with two children quoted in Grant 1996 LJMU)

Such studies show that parents in poorer households try to mitigate the effects of poverty on their children by cutting back on their own needs, as highlighted above. Middleton, *et al.* found that the study of child poverty differs when the focus is on the child or on the family and that in poorer families it may be the case that spending on children is disproportionately higher than the average (Middleton, *et al.* 1997). Children in single-parent households believed that they were worse off than children who had two parents:

> 'I'm sometimes sad, like other people get stuff and I wish I had that. Sometimes I feel like I am acting selfishly, I should be happy with what I've got.'
> (Girl, 14 years, quoted in Walker, *et al.* 2008: 434)

However for some children in single-parent households, financial support to the parent from the extended family 'buffered against any impacts of poverty' (Walker, *et al.* 2008). In terms of parental investment of time and resources in their children, living on a low income can bring some inevitable constraints. An economically deprived household will have to make some tough decisions on how they can spend some portion of their income on the purchase of books and toys, for example. It also impacts on the quality of time investment a parent can make, or whether the parent is able to emotionally disengage from the everyday difficulties of living in poverty to ensure the time spent together with children is effective and meaningful (Gershoff, *et al.* 2007). Previous studies included children younger than 11 among the respondents, with Shropshire and Middleton (1999) exploring how young people understood the economic world, as well as their immediate expectations and future desires. Children from lone-parent and income-support families worried about how their families would make ends meet. They understood and accepted that perhaps they may not get the gifts they wanted at birthdays. More importantly they failed to aspire to jobs higher than unskilled or low-paid.

In a study which compared the lives of children from different socio-economic backgrounds, Sutton (2008) highlighted how the lack of resources of estate children prevented them from engaging in alternative activities. The barriers included lack of available transport and the awareness that participation in sports or dance would cost more than their parents could afford:

'Yes leotards in our school cost £30 … you should get them for free really but you have to pay for them to be in the dance class. And it costs a lot to do the lessons, doesn't it?'

(Child quoted in Sutton 2008: 543)

Sutton also makes the point that the estate children play 'in the streets', which attracts some confrontation with local adults and police and argues that there are contradictions in government policy. Outdoor play is viewed by the government and health experts as a way in which obesity can be tackled, but the 'policing' of children within disadvantaged communities limits the areas of play or demonizes playing as being anti-social. Sutton puts forward the view that because of their social backgrounds and their 'visibility', these children tend to receive more societal disapproval than do children from different backgrounds.

Educational achievement and opportunities

Being in poverty and having diminished educational opportunities are inextricably linked. How well a child performs at school often reflects their family income, socio-economic status and class background. Children from homes where parents have lower qualifications, hold low status jobs or are claiming benefits, and those who live in poor quality housing, in disadvantaged areas, inner cities or housing estates, are less likely to be able to transcend their background and to be able to gain good qualifications when at school. Hirsch (2007) sets out to illustrate how poverty pervades the opportunities for children who grow up in poor households, affecting every stage of their childhood from preschool to young adulthood. Children even as young as three from poorer households show marked differences in terms of their basic vocabulary (they know fewer words), are less able to recognize colours and shapes, and less able to count. The effects of their backgrounds show that even before they reach school age they are at a disadvantage in that they are nine months behind in terms of school readiness.

Children from parents with low educational achievement can be as much as 12 months behind in terms of school readiness compared to children whose parents have higher educational achievements. In each year of compulsory education the poverty gap widens. By the age of 14 children from poor households are nearly two years behind the rest (Hirsch 2007).

As children get older they may reflect on the way poverty inhibits their potential experiences – they only have to look around at their lives compared to those of their peer group. Time poverty is a key issue for children, young people and parents. Being both income poor *and* time poor may prevent children being able to spend enough quality time with a parent. This was keenly felt by children in single-parent households. A study by Walker, *et al.* (2008) explored how children coped with poverty and social exclusion. In the study a 14-year-old told the researchers of his experiences:

'I've always been broke I only get money at birthdays and Christmas maybe Easter. Nothing else really. I feel poor. I just think why did my dad left [sic]?'

(Walker, *et al.* 2008: 433)

A clear link between poverty and educational attainment is demonstrated. Being eligible or not for free school meals is also identified as an indicator which signifies differential attainment levels. At age seven only 48 per cent of those taking up free school meals had reached a certain level of attainment compared to 77 per cent of those children not eligible. Children from poorer households were less likely to achieve five passes at GCSE at grade C or higher compared to other children. In terms of ethnicity it was more likely that children from Black, Bangladeshi or Pakistani families would not achieve the same levels of higher qualifications or progress as well as others (DfES 2006).

How well a parent is educated is also a significant factor. Sylva, *et al.* (2004) found that the mother's influence on the child and her level of education had more weight on children's academic performance than the father's education levels did. Further explanations of differences in levels of achievement have been explained by Bernstein (1971) as being driven by differences in language skills, with working-class children using more basic language skills – using a language 'code' deemed to be more suitable to communicate 'practical' experiences rather than abstract thought, while middle-class children use a code which allowed them to convey abstract meaning, making it a more elaborate communication code.

Schools that have higher levels of child poverty among their pupils underachieve at school-leaving exams and generally have fewer pupils staying on in education after the minimum leaving age of 16 (Brewer and Gregg 2002). The Education Maintenance Allowance (EMA) has been in existence since 2004 and a report on a pilot area in Scotland indicates that it may be helpful in keeping older children in school as well as improving their attainment levels. The study found that the EMA had a positive, independent effect on participation and attainment in national qualifications. It also found increased participation and attainment to be significantly greater in the EMA pilot areas than in the control areas. More importantly, the EMA led to a significant rise in average attainment among the EMA target group, that is young people with low standard grade attainment (Croxford and Ozga 2005).

A key strategy of the government is to reduce social exclusion through decreasing the impact that deprivation has on educational attainment, by breaking the cycle whereby childhood disadvantage follows on into adulthood, which can often be beset by social problems (Brewer and Gregg 2002). To achieve this, government, through the Social Exclusion Unit (1999), have instigated a range of initiatives targeted at key life-stages, which include strategies to deal with homelessness among young people, teenage pregnancies, and children leaving care.

Activity 4.4.2: The effects of poverty on education

- Consider the above discussion of poverty and educational achievement.
- Read Chapter 2.2 in this volume, 'The development of speech and language: inborn or bred?'.
- Summarize the adverse effect that poverty can have on the education and career prospects on an individual.

France (2008) argues that the provision of adequate housing support for young people, which also included opportunities for independent living for young mothers, would enable young people to be treated as individuals in their own right and not as dependent on their families. He also questions the decision to pay differential minimum wages, based upon age, and asks why young people who do work are economically disadvantaged in that they are expected to be able 'get by' on less income than other adults. With the minimum wage being age-banded (from October 2008, the minimum rate for adults 22+ years is £5.73, £4.77 for those aged 18–21, and £3.53 for 16- and 17-year-olds). France (ibid.) argues that to reduce poverty among young people, abandoning the age banding would be a significant step forward. There is little chance of being able to afford to set up a home and pay rent, let alone buy accommodation, on such a meagre income.

However, since the Right to Buy policy was introduced, the quantity of affordable housing has diminished and social housing building programmes have reduced alongside the deregulation of the private sectors, which has enabled landlords to have more power over tenancy agreements. For young people under 18 years of age, the housing benefit has also been reduced. The effect of these policies has been to make it extremely difficult for young people to move away from home. For those who are homeless it presents problems for organizations trying to help find them 'move on' accommodation, thus creating tensions in the homeless hostels sector (Hennessy and Grant 2005).

While the government has now included 16- and 17-year-olds in their priority need category in the Homeless Act (2002), they have also targeted teenage parents by aiming to give teenage parents who were unable to remain in the family home a place in supervised semi-independent accommodation (ODPM 2002). Teenage pregnancy has also become a disturbing aspect of the social landscape, with the UK having the highest teenage birth rate in Western Europe (SEU 1999). Although conception rates in England have fallen for under 18s since the teenage pregnancy strategy was established in 1999, the rate increased from 2001 to 2002. Many studies show that children of teenage parents are far more likely than children of older parents to be in poverty and are also more likely to suffer unfavourable outcomes as they get older. The cycle of poverty is such that there is an increased likelihood of teenage pregnancy for those who have grown up in poverty (House of Commons Work and Pensions Select Committee 2004).

Some critics argue that while New Labour has focused on ensuring that more teenage mothers enter education, training or work to avoid 'long term social exclusion', in doing so they ignore the structural and contextual barriers the young women face in gaining inclusion. More importantly, it denies the importance of full-time mothering as a valid choice (Kidger 2004). Others argue that the concepts of poverty and inequality are increasingly becoming detached from government definitions of social exclusion. Social policies have addressed the 'condition' of exclusion by frequently placing emphasis on the disconnection of the excluded from both mainstream values and norms of society, as opposed to the marginalization from material resources and a recognition of the impact poverty has on life choices (Gillies 2005). The forms of support offered and the dominant messages in government ideology highlight both the risks and disadvantages associated with early motherhood, whereas studies undertaken with young mothers found that some believed this was a positive choice, albeit often not pre-planned. The mothers associated it with providing an opportunity to create an independent life after a period in which they experienced difficulties at home and/or at school. This offers a different perspective of transition into adulthood as opposed to only focusing on the event as a accident or unfortunate incident (Arai 2003, cited in Cooke and Owen 2007).

With child poverty taking centre stage in the government's plan to tackle social exclusion, youth poverty has not had the same kind of response. According to Furlong and Cartmel (2007), NEETs are the new underclass – young people who do work are often hit hard by the government's arbitrary decision that young people can get by on a pecuniary pittance and less income than other people. Research into youth poverty has yet to fully explore the privations, experiences and nuances of the topic. However, research is beginning to tackle some key issues. The difficulties of being a normal teenager grow-ing up into adulthood and dealing with feelings of inadequacy, being accepted or not by peers and wanting to 'belong' are made more acute when living in poverty and having to deal with not always being able to have the same experiences as other children. Some researchers entered into discourses with young people and found a great deal of maturity and resignation to, and acceptance of, diminished life chances. Ridge (2002) found that teenagers were able to articulate well the privations of poverty and how it affected them. This acceptance of a lesser life and an understanding of how to live within its confines has resonance with the seminal study on the culture of poverty, where Lewis argues that 'by the age of six or seven, [they] have ... absorbed the basic attitudes and values of their subculture'. Finally, the children are written off by Lewis as being 'psychologically unready to take advantage of changing conditions or improving opportunities that may develop during their lifetime' (Lewis 1966: 5). In a 2005 UK study the experiences of youth transition outcomes in poor neighbourhoods were heavily biased, due to low or no educational attainment in the area of residence. McDonald, *et al.* (2005) acknowledged that cultural factors existed among socially excluded young adults and as such could be viewed as perpetuating, or as part of the explanation of, persistent poverty, perhaps reminiscent of Lewis's work in the 1960s. On the 'culture' exposed by Lewis, Valencia (1997) writes that 'The anti-intellectual nature of the culture of poverty and its basic lack of future orientation prohibited academic or economic success'. Breaking into the cycle through the use of education is the key to turning a young life around and doing so affects future generations.

The persistence of poverty across generations

A study by Blanden and Gibbon (2006) which compared teenagers from the 1970s with those from the 1980s found that poverty had persisted across the lifecycle. Being poor at age 16 increased the chances of children being poor when they reached their thirties. As with more recent studies the effects of being in poverty when in your teens are perhaps more to do with where you live, whether your parents are employed or not and whether your parents have a good standard of education (Blanden and Gibbon 2006).

The British system of education was changed in 1972 to ensure that all children stayed on in school until 16 years of age. The post-16 education system was designed to enable the more able to remain in education until 18 and access to continued learning became free up to the age of 18. The state would provide adult education for those who sought it, with no special treatment or targeting of specific groups. Yet when faced with the evidence, it could be argued that the system worked against equality of opportunity. Forsyth and Furlong (2000) found that despite having similar educational attainment to others, disadvantaged children were still less likely to enter higher education. This cycle of poverty has been found in studies which have examined cohorts of teenagers in the past and tracked their progress into later life.

When the school leaving age was raised to sixteen this had the effect of improving the opportunities of young people from poorer backgrounds and lower achievers. In an analysis of the economic advantages 'staying on' at school had, it was found to raise wages by 10 per cent, compared to the wages of those who did not do the extra year (Dickson 2008). Hence there is a strong argument, on efficiency grounds, to improve the education participation of groups who are at risk of poor attainment and life chances. Evidence from the evaluation of EMAs would suggest that paying young people to stay on at school has made a positive impact on preventing some young people entering the NEET group. However, the EMA was less successful in attracting young people back into full-time education once they had entered the NEET group.

Getting some GCSEs, albeit at lower grades, will allow for access to further learning. However, for those young people who obtain few or no qualifications at 16 their opportunities diminish and they are likely to leave school with much poorer prospects. Despite efforts to improve qualifications of young people there has been little change in the number of young people who leave school without qualifications. This helps to explain why there have been no significant reductions in the numbers of NEETs who are not participating in education, employment or training in their late teens. The UK has one of the highest percentages of NEETs – only four out of 21 other OECD countries have higher rates (UNICEF 2007).

The transitionary period between childhood and adulthood is now somewhat blurred; in the post-welfare state UK many young people entered work from the age of 15, notably those from the baby boom years, and by the age of 18 would have had three years of employment behind them. They felt 'grown up', had a sense of purpose and for many a sense of responsibility and desire to help out their parents. Although 16- to 18-year-olds receive some policy attention in that they are required to participate in school, training or work-related experiences until the age of 18, the choices open to them seem to be diminishing. The Department for Education and Skills will tackle the problem of young people with inadequate qualifications or skills by raising 'participation' levels: raising the school-leaving age from 16 (set in 1972) to 18 in 2013 (students do not necessarily have to stay in school but can undergo training or work placements) (DCSF 2007). In a report published by the Princes Trust the personal cost of not participating in either education training or work was estimated to impose a wage scar on an individual of between 8 and 15 per cent (2007). MacDonald, *et al.* (2005) found that many young males had already experienced a chequered training/work history and had tried various government schemes – which rarely translated into long-term or lasting employment – that led to low-level, low-paid work that often left them feeling marginalized, on the outside looking in. These groups were very often made up of young people from the most deprived areas of the UK who had failed to achieve in the education system, now either languishing in the poorly paid jobs market, or in the ranks of the unemployed, or NEETs.

The problem of youth poverty has been marginalized and is now receiving similar treatment to the feckless poor of Rowntree's era in that youths (often perceived as males) are more visible, especially in urban areas. Negative perceptions of hoodies hanging around the streets serve to demonize them and provide fodder for the alienation of this marginalized group. For those who do not have the support at home or the motivation to succeed in school or college, the long-term prospects may be bleak unless the measures designed to break the cycle of disadvantage or missed opportunities can be changed.

Student reflection

Review your responses to Activity 4.4.1 and consider the following:

- How does living in a household affected by poverty impact upon children's lives?
- Drawing from your own experiences or observations, in what way can poverty affect the educational experience of young people?

Key points

- Child poverty today differs from poverty at the beginning of the century in that children in the UK are not allowed to work today, and there exists greater inequality of opportunity for young people.
- There is disagreement as to whether/how poverty exists today in Britain which influences the ways of addressing it.
- Lack of money makes it harder for children to take part in and enjoy activities with friends and/or maintain friendships, resulting in social exclusion and adverse affects on their future opportunities.
- Household location, composition and characteristics, and whether parents are in receipt of benefits are key factors in identifying poverty.
- New Labour's anti-poverty strategy has been to address child poverty (0–15) with a number of key policies: support for parents to work, financial support, improvement in public services and the improvement of parenting skills.
- Issues surround the measurement of child poverty. Evidence suggests that relative spending on children can be similar or even higher than in more affluent households, with parents cutting back on themselves. However 'time poverty' involving the amount of quality time children have with a parent and the issues surrounding the language skills of 'poor' children on entry to education are important factors in socialization of children.
- There have been some attempts to address the social inequalities resulting from child poverty, such as a minimum wage and housing support, however these are significantly lower for the 16–17 and 18–21 age groups.
- The educational attainments of disadvantaged children are often far lower than those who are not socially disadvantaged and those who manage to attain good results are less likely to enter higher education. That said, there is evidence to suggest that a way of overcoming poverty is to improve the educational participation of 'at risk' groups.

Note

1   Since 2004–5 the Family Resources Survey (FRS), from which most of the government's measures of childhood poverty are drawn, has collected data on material deprivation.

Recommended reading

Alcock, P. (1993) *Understanding Poverty*, London: Macmillan.
Brewer, M. and Gregg, P. (2002) *Eradicating Child Poverty in Britain: Welfare Reform and Children Since 1997*, Working Paper 02/052, Centre for Market and Public Organisation, Bristol: Department of Economics, University of Bristol.
Levitas, R. (1998) *The Inclusive Society? Social Exclusion and New Labour*, London: Macmillan.
Thane, P. (1982) *The Foundations of the Welfare State: Social Policy in Modern Britain*, London: Longman.

References

Alcock, P. (1993) *Understanding Poverty*, 2nd edn, London: Macmillan.
Bernstein, B. (1971) *Class Codes and Control: Vol. 1*, London: Routledge and Kegan Paul.
Blair, T. (1999) Beveridge revisited: A welfare state for the 21st century, in R. Walker (ed.) *Ending Child Poverty: Popular Welfare for the 21st Century?* Bristol: Policy Press.
Boardman, B. (1992) *Fuel Poverty*, London: Belhaven Press.

Bradbury, B. and Jäntti, M. (1999) Child poverty across industrialized countries, *Journal of Population and Social Security (Population)*, Supplement to Vol. 1: 385–410.

Brewer, M. and Gregg, P. (2002) Eradicating child poverty in Britain: welfare, reform and children since 1997, in Walker, R. and Wiseman, M. (eds) *The Welfare We Want*, Bristol: Policy Press.

Bradshaw (2006) *A Review of the Comparative Evidence on Child Poverty*, York: Joseph Rowntree Foundation.

Brown, G. (2004) *Speech by Gordon Brown at the Joseph Rowntree Centenary Lecture, London*, Our Children are Our Future – Joseph Rowntree Lecture, 8 July. Available online at: http://www.hm-treasury.gov.uk/press_65_04.htm

Cooke, J. and Owen, J. (2007) 'A place of our own?' Teenage mothers' views on housing needs and support models, *Children & Society*, 21: 56–68.

CPAG (2008) *Child Poverty the Stats: Analysis of the Latest Poverty Statistics*, London: CPAG, October.

Croxford, I. and Ozga, J. (2005) *Enterprise and Lifelong Learning Research Programme: Education Maintenance Allowances (EMAs) Attainment of National Qualifications in the Scottish Pilots*, Research Findings No.25/2005, Glasgow: Scottish Executive Social Research.

Department for Children, Schools and Families (DCSF) (2008) *Reducing the Number of People Classed as NEET, the Strategy*, London: DCSF.

—— (2007) *Raising the Participation Age in Education and Training to 18: Review of Existing Evidence of the Benefits and Challenges*, Research Brief No: DCSF-RB012, November, London: DCSF.

Department for Work and Pensions (DWP) (2008) *Households Below Average Income: An Analysis of the Income Distribution 1994/95–2006/07*, London: The Stationery Office.

DfES (2006) *Social Mobility: Narrowing Social Class Educational Attainment Gaps*. London: DfES.

Dickson, M. (2008) *The Causal Effect of Education on Wages Revisited*, University of Warwick mimeo.

France, A. (2008) From being to becoming: the importance of tackling youth poverty in transitions to adulthood, *Social Policy and Society*, 7: 495–505.

Forsyth, A. and Furlong, A. (2000) *Socioeconomic Disadvantage and Access to Higher Education*, York: Joseph Rowntree Foundation.

Furlong, A. and Cartmel, F. (2007) *Young People and Social Change: New Perspectives*, Maidenhead: McGraw-Hill/OUP.

Gershoff, E. T., Aber, J. L., Raver, C. and Lennon, M. C. (2007) Income is not enough: incorporating material hardship into models of income associations with parenting and child development, *Child Development*, 78 (1): 70–95.

Gibbons, S. and Blanden, J. (2006) *The Persistence of Poverty Across Generations: A View from Two British Cohorts*. Bristol: Polity Press.

Gillies, V. (2005) Meeting parents' needs? Discourses of 'support' and 'inclusion' in family policy, *Critical Social Policy*, 25; 70.

Goode, J., Callender, C. and Lister, R. (1998) *Purse or Wallet? Gender Inequalities and Income Distribution within Families on Benefits*, London: Policy Studies Institute.

Gordon, D., Adelman, L., Ashworth, K., Bradshaw, J., Levitas, R., Middleton, S., Pantazis, C., Patsios, D., Payne, S., Townsend, P. and Williams, J. (2000) *Poverty and Social Exclusion in Britain*, York: Joseph Rowntree Foundation.

Grant, D. K. (1996) Poverty in Britain in the 1990s: Rowntree revisited, PhD Thesis, Liverpool: John Moores University.

Grant, D. K., Maxwell, S. (1998) Food coping strategies: a century on from Rowntree, *Nutrition and Health*, 13: 45–60.

Hennessy, C. and Grant, D. (2005) Young and homeless: an evaluation of a resettlement service on Merseyside, *International Journal of Consumer Studies*, 29 (2): 137–47.

—— (2006) *Gender Discrimination and Ageist Perceptions Training Initiative: Evaluation Report*, Liverpool: Liverpool John Moores University.

Hidden Lives: online at http://www.hiddenlives.org.uk (maintained by the Children's Society).

Hirsch, D. (2007) Chicken and Egg: Child Poverty and Educational Inequalities – *CPAG Policy Briefing*, London: CPAG, September.

House of Commons Work and Pensions Select Committee (2004), *Child Poverty in the UK*, Second Report, Session 2003–4, HC 85, London: The Stationery Office.

Iavacou, M. and Berthoud, R (2006) *The Economic Position of Large Families*, Department for Work and Pensions Research Report No. 358, Leeds: Corporate Document Services. London: The Stationery Office.

Kidger, J. (2004) Supporting Teenage Parents Including Young Mothers: limitations to New Labour's strategy for supporting teenage parents. *Critical Social Policy*, 24: 291.

Leather, S. (1992) Less money, less choice?, in National Consumer Council (eds) *Your Food: Whose Choice?*, London: HMSO.

Lewis, O. (1966) The culture of poverty, *Scientific American*, 215 (4): 3–10.

Lister, R. Povertyism and 'othering': why they matter. A talk by Professor Ruth Lister at the TUC conference, 'Challenging Poverty – the Media and Politicians', Brighton, 17 October 2008.

Lloyd, E. (2006) Children, poverty and social exclusion, in C. Pantazis, D. Gordon and R. Levitas (eds) *Poverty and Social Exclusion in Britain: The Millennium Survey*, Bristol: Policy Press.

Mack, J. and Lansley, S. (1985) *Poor Britain*, London and Boston: George Allen and Unwin.

Magadi, M. and Middleton, S. (2007) *Severe Child Poverty in the UK*, London: Save the Children. Available online at: http://www.crsp.ac.uk/downloads/publications/bpc/severe_child_poverty_in_the_uk.pdf

McDonald, R., Shildrick, T., Webster, C. and Simpson D. (2005) Growing up in poor neighbourhoods: the significance of class and place in the extended transistions of 'socially excluded' young adults, *Sociology* 39 (5): 873–91.

Middleton, S., Ashworth, K. and Braithwaite, I. (1997) *Small Fortunes: Spending on Children, Childhood Poverty and Parental Sacrifice*, York: Joseph Rowntree Foundation.

Moore, J. (1989) 'The end of the line for poverty', speech to the Greater London Area CPC, 11 May.

ODPM (2002) *Good Practice in Supported Housing for Young Mothers*, London: ODPM.

Piachaud, D (1979) *The Cost of a Child*, London: CPAG.

Platt, L. (2007) *Poverty and Ethnicity in the UK*, 1st edn, Bristol: Policy Press.

The Princes Trust (2007) *The Cost of Exclusion: Counting the Cost of Youth Disadvantage in the UK*. Available online at: http://www.princes-trust.org.uk/PDF/ (accessed 14 August 2009).

Ridge, T. (2002) *Childhood Poverty and Social Exclusion: From a Child's Perspective*, Bristol: Policy Press.

Rowntree, B. S. (1901) *Poverty: A Study of Town Life*, London: Macmillan and Co.

—— (1937) *The Human Needs of Labour*, 2nd edn, London: Longmans, Green and Co.

Rowntree, B. S. and Lavers, G.R. (1951) *Poverty and the Welfare State: A Third Social Survey of York Dealing only with Economic Questions*, London: Longmans, Green and Co.

Sayer, A. (2005) Class, moral worth and recognition, *Sociology*, 39 (5): 947–63.

Shropshire, J. and Middleton, S. (1999) *Small Expectations: Learning to be Poor?*, York: Joseph Rowntree Foundation.

Social Exclusion Unit (1999) *Teenage Pregnancy*, London: The Stationery Office, June.

Stitt, S. and Grant, D. (1993) *Poverty: Rowntree Re-visited*, Aldershot: Avebury Press.

Sutton, L. (2008) The state of play: disadvantage, play and children's well-being, *Social Policy and Society*, 7 (4): 537–49. Sylva, K., Melhuish, E., Sammons, O, Siraj-Blatchford, I. and Taggart, B. (2004) *The Effective Provision of Pre-school Education (EPPE) Project: Findings from the early Primary Years*, London: DfES.

Sylva, K., Melhuish, E., Sammons, O., Siraj-Blatchford, I. and Taggart, B. (2004) *The Effective Provision of Pre-school Education (EPPE) Project: Findings from the Early Primary Years*, London: DfES.

Thane, P. (1982) *The Foundations of the Welfare State: Social Policy in Modern Britain*, London: Longman.

The Children's Society (2008) *Living on the Edge of Despair: Destitution amongst Asylum Seeking and Refugee Children*, Childhood Destitution Report Summary, London: The Children's Society.

UNICEF (2007) *Child Poverty in Perspective: An Overview of Child Well-being in Rich Countries*, Florence: UNICEF Innocenti Research Centre.

Valencia, R. (1997) *The Evolution of Deficit Thinking: Educational Thought and Practice*, London: Routledge.

Veit-Wilson, J. (1998) *Setting Adequacy Standards*, Bristol: Policy Press.

Walker, J., Crawford, K. and Taylor, F. (2008) Listening to children: gaining a perspective of the experiences of poverty and social exclusion from children and young people of single parent families, *Health and Social Care in the Community*, 16 (4): 429–36.

West, A. (2007) Poverty and educational achievement: why do children from low income families tend to do less well at school?, *Benefits*, 15 (3): 283–97.

Part 5

The global child

The final part of this book looks at childhood and issues facing children and young people within a broader, more global context.

The first chapter by Qouta, focusing on the experiences of children living in Palestine, explores the effect of living in a war zone and experiencing trauma on children's mental health. Qouta points out that until fairly recently there had been little research carried out on either children's experiences of conflict based trauma or in general on the experiences of people living through the conflict in Palestine.

The chapter highlights the negative impact that trauma can have on children resulting in post traumatic stress disorder (PTSD) which can last into adolescence and adulthood. Although the focus is on the Gaza Strip, the chapter is important for those working with and treating children suffering from PTSD anywhere in the world.

Torstensson's chapter explores the impact on children of living with the HIV/AIDS epidemic in sub-Saharan Africa. The chapter highlights how living within this context affects children, not only those born suffering from the disease or those who are orphaned by the disease, but all children within the area. Having AIDS in the family or living within an area plighted by the epidemic can induce fear and anxiety about the future, such as being orphaned, having to care for the family and deal with everyday life. These fears and anxieties can impact strongly on the psychological and emotional well-being of the children. Torstensson points out that, in the absence of a cure for the disease, it is vital that we listen to the children living through the pandemic in order to empower them to become agents of change.

The final chapter of the book explores the experiences of children and young people who migrate for work and/or for education within the Developing or Majority world. Punch begins by pointing out that most literature on child refugees focuses on the negative experience of those who are coerced by parents to migrate for economic reasons, or those who are trafficked and exploited as child slaves or prostitutes. Punch states that, in reality, many children migrate of their own volition in order to improve their lives and the lives of their families through seeking better employment and/or educational opportunities. In fact, Punch highlights the fact that in some communities migration is part of the culture and for young people it can be a rite of passage into maturity.

Punch explores the benefits that young people can gain from migration such as economic reward, broadening of horizons, improved future prospects and gaining respect from family and peers, as well as the negative experiences they may have such as homesickness, poor working conditions and physical or sexual abuse.

Punch states that as there are many misconceptions concerning the reasons for child migration and the experiences they have as refugees, it is important to listen to them and their perceptions of migration. She concludes that while many children choose to migrate we must remember that their choices are often very limited and the choice to migrate may merely constitute the better choice among a set of poor options, such as poverty, lack of future prospects and possibly death.

5.1 The Palestinian experience
Brutalized childhoods

Samir Qouta

Warfare and trauma

Researchers and scientists concerned with the consequences of trauma on children's mental health disagree about its impact, but they agree that there is not a linear correlation between trauma and children's mental health.

Clinical research conducted during the Second World War showed both unexpected resilience (Bordman 1944; Freud and Burlingham 1942) and marked psychological disturbances among civilians, especially children (Dundson 1941; Glover 1942; Janis 1951; Rachman 1978). While relatively few psychological disorders have been documented during actual wartime, an increase in post-traumatic stress disorders (PTSDs) is well documented among soldiers (Figley 1985; Horowitz 1985), concentration camp survivors (Eitinger 1973; Shanan 1989) and political prisoners (Foster, *et al.* 1987).

Studies of contemporary wars also tend to show that exposure to political violence does not directly increase psychological distress. Studies on riots in Northern Ireland have reported, in general, few mental health problems (Fee 1980; Fraser 1971; McAuley and Troy 1983; Cairns and Wilson 1989). However, in a study conducted ten years after the beginning of the riots, Cairns and Wilson (1984) found a positive relationship between residing in a high tension area and psychological distress. Similarly, although research on the Beirut population immediately after the Israeli invasion showed no increase in mental health problems (Hourani, *et al.* 1986), two years after the invasion a remarkable increase in psychological distress and especially in psychosomatic problems among children was found (Rayhid, *et al.* 1986).

This chapter reports on research carried out into the effects of conflict in Palestine on the mental health of children, although some reference is made to impact on adults. The research provided an opportunity to expand the knowledge base regarding long-term, community-wide trauma and highlights effective ways to serve those in the society, particularly children who are suffering from conflict-related trauma.

Studies summarized here investigated the relationship between trauma and cognitive/emotional responses; collective punishment and its effect on mental health; and the prevalence of PTSD among mothers and children who had been exposed to shelling and/or loss of their homes.

Activity 5.1.1: Children and trauma

- Make a list of those aspects, events and effects of conflict that you feel might traumatise a child.
- What might be the long-term consequences of this, in terms of the behaviour, emotional development and life chances of children traumatized in these ways?

Trauma and children's mental health in the Palestinian context

The Palestinian context

The research reported here began in 1990, in the middle of the first popular uprising against the ongoing Israeli military occupation of the Gaza Strip and West Bank which continues today in the form of the second Intifada. The first Intifada lasted from 1987 to roughly 1993, when the Oslo Peace Accords were signed. Between 1993 and 2000 the 'facts on the ground' did not change for those living in the Palestinian Occupied Territories, despite the hope and promise embedded in the Peace Accords. Many Palestinians continued to live with poverty, violent repression of political activity, lack of access to water, increasing settlement building in the territories by the Israeli Government (and concomitant expulsion of Palestinians), and no control over their own borders. After seven years of what many Palestinians construed as empty promises, the second Intifada began.

In September of 2000, the then Knesset member Ariel Sharon visited the Muslim holy place Haram Al-Sharif, or Temple Mount, with a large contingent of armed guards. As he is viewed by many as an aggressor towards Palestinian refugees in Lebanon, this act was interpreted as an aggressive incitement by those holding this view. During Muslim prayers the following day, many Palestinian citizens of Israel protested the visit. The crowd was shot into with live rounds, resulting in the death and injury of many. And thus, the second Intifada was born. This Intifada has been far more violent than the first, with demolition of homes and farms and tighter restrictions on entering and leaving the Gaza Strip resulting in roughly 600 Israeli deaths and 3,250 Palestinian deaths (Palestinian Center for Human Rights).

Trauma and children

A traumatic event, as defined by the Royal College of Psychiatrists (http://www.rcpsych.ac.uk) is one where we can see that we are in danger, our life is threatened, or where we see other people dying or being injured. The event may range from a road accident to violent personal assault and, as stated above, it may cause trauma to those involved in the event, as well as those witnessing it.

One of the conditions most closely associated with exposure to traumatic events is the anxiety disorder, PTSD. The term PTSD is somewhat of an umbrella term and may involve emotional responses such as depression, grief, guilt and anger and physical responses such as muscle aches and pains, headaches, exhaustion and even diarrhoea. People suffering from PTSD often experience flashbacks and nightmares, which rob them of their sleep, and/or hypervigilance, a sense of being on guard or continually looking for and expecting trouble, which again can lead to exhaustion.

Research by Thabet, *et al.* (2002) and Thabet and Vostanis (1998) has highlighted the fact that trauma does not take place in a vacuum but in a certain community and in a certain historical context. Both studies found significant evidence of increased mental ill health, depression, anxiety, sleeping difficulties symptomatic of PTSD among children living in conditions of warfare and military violence.

Research by Qouta, *et al.* (1995) found that between 20 and 25 per cent of children living through conflict in the Gaza Strip suffered from PTSD, which is comparable with the levels of PTSD found among Israeli and Lebanese children by Laor, *et al.* (1997) and Saigh (1991) respectively. However, a later study conducted by Qouta, *et al.* (2003) during the second Intifada revealed an increased level – between 58 and 65 per cent of PTSD among children. This evidence implies a direct correlation between levels of violence and PTSD in children for, as noted above, the second Intifada has been more violent than the first (Palestinian Center for Human Rights). In fact, a community survey by Abu Hein, *et al.* (1993) of 1,200 Gazan children aged seven to 15 years of age revealed that 92.5 per cent had been tear-gassed, 85 per cent has been subjected to night raids, 55 per cent had witnessed assaults on family members, 42 per cent had been beaten, 23 per cent had been injured and 19 per cent had been detained. There is hardly any wonder that a majority of these children suffered from PTSD.

Palestinian children and research

Although much has been written about the Palestinians, little attention has been given to the study of Palestinian children. This deficiency becomes even more apparent when one looks for empirical investigations of children in the occupied territories. Palestinian children first became the subjects of serious academic research in the early 1980s, when Punamäki began to study the influence of the occupation on the mental health of children. It is interesting to note that initial academic efforts to study Palestinian children were carried out by non-Palestinians.

The relatively limited research on Palestinian children can be attributed to many factors. In the first place, there is a lack of experienced local researchers. The number of qualified and trained Palestinian researchers is extremely limited and, although this scarcity is evident throughout the various disciplines, it is particularly acute in the social sciences. This shortage is partially due to the lack of institutions of higher learning in the occupied territories, especially at the graduate level. Palestinian universities did not come into being until the mid-1980s.

Secondly, there have been restrictions on research in the occupied territories. Israel has not sanctioned academic research without prior consent. Many felt that this violates principles of academic freedom and a few Palestinians risked conducting research openly.

Finally, there is reluctance among the population to participate in research. The daily difficulties experienced by the local population under occupation naturally precluded co-operation with strangers. People were generally hesitant to divulge information to others for fear that it would be used against them. They feared the police and Israeli intelligence (Baker 1990).

Children, conflict and trauma: the research

The first serious empirical research carried out by Palestinian investigators was in the form of the studies conducted by Baker (1990), Baker, *et al.* (1991) and Khamis (1993;

1995). These studies found that the children involved suffered from a high frequency of nightmares, enuresis (bed-wetting), anxiety and aggressive behaviour – all symptoms of PTSD.

Khamis (1993) was interested particularly in the presence of PTSD in young males injured during the Intifada, in its development and in the factors affecting adjustment. She found that for those suffering from PTSD the perceived social support did not act as an antidote, although it did facilitate adjustment.

In her second study (Khamis 1995) Khamis included females and participants of all ages. She found that the passage of time did not improve the ability of the individual to psychologically adjust to society. Trauma studies, in general, find that a person's capability to adjust correlates positively with a set of situational variables such as social support and special care, whereas it is negatively affected by injury and related variables such as visible deformities. It is likely that the severity and visibility of an injury increases the difficulty of assimilating the trauma because they promote negative self-concepts, frustration, concern about stigma, feelings of dependency and disapproval from the environment. In this research, Khamis found that single people and those with more education were better adjusted, whereas adolescents were less well adjusted and less able to initiate and maintain social relationships. One can assume that recognizing the variables which compound PTSD is essential in effective treatment of the disorder.

Baker (1990) surveyed Palestinian children from the perspective of their physical health and their socio-economic, psychological and pedagogical states. He found unusually high levels of conduct and sleep disorder, as well as fear. Some of them did not perform at the expected level on some Piagetian tasks and drop-out from school was high, especially for females. The enforced closure of schools seemed to have had a negative effect from an educational, psychosocial and cognitive perspective. Surprisingly, he found that Palestinian children displayed higher levels of self-esteem and a more internal locus of control compared with other Arab children.

In his second study, Baker (Baker *et al.* 1991) surveyed Palestinian children who had been subjected to violence. Violent, destructive and self-destructive behaviour as well as headaches and sleep disorders appeared to be very common among them. Nevertheless, they had high levels of self-esteem.

Punamäki (1984; 1987a; 1987b; 1990) conducted studies in which she explored the effects of violence and the military occupation on Palestinian children. She found that fear, withdrawal, sleep difficulties and nightmares were common and that 80 per cent of the children involved in the studies were afraid that the Israeli army would attack their home.

Punamäki (1990) was concerned with discovering which psychological and social factors could mitigate the negative impact on mental health of hardships such as exposure to violence. She found that while experience of political violence did increase active and courageous behaviour in children, this was not able to mitigate the negative impact of extreme hardships on their mental health. The only factor which could protect children's mental health was their mother's firm belief in the national cause.

Research such as that of Pynoos and Eth (1985) indicates that there is no linear relationship between exposure to political violence or war and psychological disorders. If disorders occur, they often are delayed and appear in veiled forms. This result can be understood as an indication of the endurance, competence and creativity of the human psyche, and as evidence of the numerous psychological processes and social factors which mitigate the negative impact of political violence on mental health. People are not passive victims of their environment but rather they are employers of vital resources in the construction and maintenance of their integrity and psychological stability.

Qouta, *et al.* (1995) conducted a study which aimed to build a comprehensive picture of the relationship between political violence and the cognitive capacity and emotional well-being of children. They found that the relationship between Intifada-related traumatic events and psychological responses depended on whether the child was a passive or an active participant in traumatic events.

The cognitive capacity of the children was assessed by measuring intelligence, creativity, concentration and memory. Neuroticism, self-esteem and risk-taking were used as indicators of emotional well-being. It was predicted that the relationship between traumatic experiences and cognitive capacity would be mediated through the emotional maturity of the child, and that emotional health is affected by cognitive capacity.

The researchers had two competing and contrasting hypotheses:

- Traumatic experience disturbs healthy functioning of cognitive capacity.
- The challenge of trauma improves the children's cognitive capacity.

The results of the study confirmed the fact that there is not a linear correlation between experience of trauma and psychological impact and, to some degree, confirmed both of the hypotheses above.

In the first place, in relation to the first hypothesis, the study suggested that traumatic experience does constitute a risk factor for children's cognitive capabilities. However, evidence indicated that the impact of the trauma depended on two variables.

The first variable was the actual nature of the cognitive function being investigated as not all aspects of cognitive capability were affected in the same way by trauma. Secondly, the level of exposure to traumatic experiences and/or the level of participation in the violence impacted on cognitive functioning.

In terms of response to trauma, the cognitive capabilities measured seemed to divide into two groups. Intelligence, creativity, visio-motor performance and ability to organize symbolic material were not affected by trauma, whether or not the children had been exposed to a low level or a high level of traumatic experiences or whether or not they had participated in the violence. On the other hand, the impact of trauma on concentration, attention and memory varied. When children had been passive or exposed to a low number of traumatic experiences, concentration, attention and memory were negatively affected. However, in children who had been exposed to a high number of traumatic events or who had actually participated in the violence, there were fewer problems with concentration, attention and memory.

The results led Qouta, *et al.* (1995) to suggest that, as active participation in trauma was related to fewer concentration, attention and memory problems, perhaps the second hypothesis given above – that the challenge of trauma improves the children's cognitive capacity – is true to some extent.

Student reflection

In view of the impact that violence has on children, to what extent might it be considered a war crime for states not to take into consideration the needs of children when conducting military operations in predominately civilian areas? Do military organisations have a duty of care towards children?

They concluded that this non-linear affect of trauma on the cognitive abilities of children has important implications for school performance and post-traumatic treatment and that an understanding of it is beneficial to professionals working with children in war zones or ex-war zones.

In terms of emotional response to trauma, the results of this study confirmed that exposure to political traumatic experiences, such as violence, humiliation, and loss of family members, increases children's psychological suffering. The highest level of neuroticism was found among active boys who were exposed to many traumatic experiences. While increased neuroticism and risk-taking were found among the Palestinian children studied, children's active participation in the Intifada could not protect children from developing emotional problems, as was originally assumed.

Within war zones and conflict situations, what are termed 'collective punishments' are frequently imposed upon those under occupation. Research has considered the consequences on the mental health of children and young people in the Gaza Strip of the 'collective punsihments' of curfews and home destruction.

During the first Intifada, citizens of the Gaza Strip had a nightly curfew and occasionally random curfews were enforced during the day time. Under curfew, all aspects of daily life are paralyzed and this can result in the breakdown of normal patterns of social, intimate and economic interactions. Parents expressed strong worry about the impact of constant curfews on children's well-being and behaviour, and research conducted by Qouta and El Sarraj (1992) concurred with them. The results of this research showed that 66 per cent of children fought with each other more than before the curfew, 54 per cent were afraid of new things, 38 per cent developed aggressive behaviour, 19 per cent suffered from bed-wetting, and 2.3 per cent began to have speech difficulties.

Qouta, *et al.* (1996) conducted research which compared the psychological distress of parents and children who had lost their homes with those who had witnessed the destruction of houses and with a control group who neither had their homes destroyed nor witnessed the destruction of homes.

A house is not only a shelter, it is a home and, as such, can be the heart of family life embedded with memories and attachment to familiar objects, and feelings of security and consolation. Thus the destruction of a home can be a very painful and traumatic experience. The United Nations (UN 2005) calculated that between 2000 and 2004 nearly 12,000 Palestinian houses on the West Bank were damaged and of them 4,000 were completely destroyed. Qouta, *et al.* (1996) found that parents, especially mothers, who lost their homes showed a higher level of anxiety, depression and paranoiac symptoms than witnesses and parents in the control group. Of children who had lost their homes, 60 per cent suffered from symptoms of PTSD, intrusive re-experiencing, withdrawal symptoms, and night terrors. In the witness group the symptoms varied between 28–41 per cent and in the control group between 4–12 per cent. The results thus indicate that merely witnessing violence targeted at others can form a risk for child mental health.

There are other factors of life in a war zone which can impact on the mental health of children in a negative way, such as restricted movement of citizens, which can prevent or delay parent–child interaction. Qouta, *et al.* (2006) report that longitudinal studies provided evidence that childhood traumatic stress can result in increased psychological distress and decreased positive resources in adolescents. Moreover, high exposure to military trauma in middle childhood can lead to prolonged sufferance from PTSD in adulthood.

Conclusion

It is a tragic fact that Palestinian children have become laboratories for the study of the relationship between trauma and violence, conflict, and children's well-being during war. Wars and battles have been fought without interruption in the region for more than 50 years. None of these wars, however, has brought a solution to the conflict between Jews and Arabs and the atmosphere of insecurity, danger, violence, and hostility that prevails during the violent periods has inevitably left scars on the mental health of Palestinian children. It can only be hoped that the lessons learned from this situation concerning children's mental health can be beneficial to children everywhere who experience trauma.

Student reflection

- What might the research discussed in this chapter teach us about how to treat children suffering from mental health issues due to traumatic experiences?

Key points

- Research has shown that living through traumatic experiences such as those experienced in war zones can result in mental health problems, in particular post-traumatic stress disorder (PTSD).
- There has been brutal and bloody conflict in Palestine, particularly on the Gaza Strip, for many years and this has had an effect on the mental health of people living there.
- The levels of children suffering from PTSD in Palestine increased markedly during the second Intifada.
- Prior to the 1980s little was written about Palestinian children due to the fact that there were few experienced researchers in Palestine. The Israeli Government had to sanction all research and also the Palestinian people were often afraid of divulging information for fear of reprisals.
- Research has shown that there is no linear correlation between mental health issues and exposure to violence and warfare.
- Exposure to violence can affect cognitive capabilities in terms of concentration, attention and memory, but not in terms of intelligence, creativity, visio-motor performance and the ability to organize symbolic material.
- Participation in the violence – rather than being a passive victim of it – can in fact reduce the negative impact on mental health.
- Such experiences as the destruction of one's home, curfews and the restriction of movement that often occur during warfare can also impact on mental health negatively.

Recommended reading

Beah, I. (2007) *A Long Way Gone: Memoirs of a Boy Soldier*, London: Fourth Estate.
Booth, N., Strang, A. and Wessells, M. (2006) *A World Turned Upside Down: Social Ecological Approaches to Children in War Zone*, New York: Kumarian Press.
Ellis, D. (2007) *Three Wishes: Palestinian and Isreali Children Speak*, New York: Frances Lincoln Publishers.
Machel, G. (2001) *The Impact of War on Children: A Review of Progress Since the 1996 United Nations Report on the Impact of Armed Conflict on Chidlren*, London: Hurst and Co. Publishers Ltd.

References

Abu Hein, F., Qouta, S., Thabet, A. and El Sarraj, E. (1993) Truama and the mental health of children in Gaza, *British Medical Journal*, 306: 1130–1.

Baker, A. (1990) Psychological responses of Palestinian children to the environmental stress associated with military occuptaion, *Journal of Refugee Studies*, 4: 237–47.

Baker, A., El Husseini, S., Arafat, C. and Ajush, D. (1991) *The Palestinian Child in the West Bank and Gaza Strip*, Jerusalem: El Tawin Institution (in Arabic).

Bordman, F. (1944) Child psychiatry in wartime Britain, *Journal of Educational Psychology*, 35: 293–301.

Cairns, E. and Wilson, R. (1984) The impact of political violence on mild psychiatric morbidity in Northern Ireland, *British Journal of Psychiatry*, 145: 631–4.

—— (1989) Mental health aspects of political violence in Northern Ireland, *International Journal of Mental Health*, 18, 38–56.

Dundson, M. I. (1941) A psychologist's contribution to air raid problems, *Mental Health*, 2: 37–41.

Eitinger, L. (1973) Mental diseases among refugees in Norway after World War II, in C. A. Zwingmann and A. Pfister-Ammende (eds) *Uprooting and After*, New York: Springer-Verlag.

Fee, F. (1980) Responses to a behavioural questionnaire of a group of Belfast children, in J. Harbison and J. Harbison (eds) *A Society under Stress: Children and Young People in Northern Ireland*, Somerset: Open Books.

Figley, C. R. (1985) *Trauma and its Wake: The Study and Treatment of Post-traumatic Stress Disorder*, New York: Brunner/Mazel.

Fraser, R. M. (1971) The cost of commotion: an analysis of the psychiatric sequel of the 1969 Belfast riots, *British Journal of Psychiatry*, 118: 257–64.

Foster, D., Davis, D. and Sandler, D. (1987) *Detention and Torture in South Africa. Psychological legal and historical studies*, Cape Town: Davis Phillip

Freud, A. and Burlingham, D. (1942) *Young Children in Wartime*, London: Allen & Unwin.

—— (1943) *War and Children*, New York: Ernest Willard.

Glover, E. (1942) Notes on the psychological effects of war conditions on the civilian population, *International Journal of Psychoanalysis*, 23: 17–37.

Hourani, L., Armenian, H., Zuryk, H. and Afifi, L. (1986) A population-based survey of loss and psychological distress during war, *Social Science and Medicine*, 23, 269–75.

Horowitz, M. J. (1985) Disasters and psychological responses to stress, *Psychiatric Annals*, 15: 161–4.

Janis, I. (1951) *Air War and Emotional Stress*, New York: McGraw-Hill.

Khamis, V. (1993) Victims of the Intifada: the psychosocial adjustment of the injured, *Behavioral Medicine*, 19: 93–101.

—— (1995) Psychological sequels of Intifada-related trauma in Palestinian families, unpublished manuscript, Bethlehem University.

Laor, N., Wolmer, L., and Cohen, D. J. (2001) Mothers' functioning and children's symptoms 5 years after a scud missile attack, *The American Journal of Psychiatry*, 158: 1020–6.

Laor, N., Wolmer, L., Mayes, L., Gershon, A., Weizman, R. and Cohen, D. (1997) Israeli Preschool Children Under Scuds: A 30-Month Follow-up, *Journal of the American Academy of Child & Adolescent Psychiatry*, 36 (3): 349–56.

Lynons, H. A. (1971) Psychiatric sequel of the Belfast Riots. *British Journal of Psychiatry*, 118: 257–64.

McAuley, R. and Troy, M. (1983) The impact of urban conflict and violence on children referred to a child psychiatric clinic, in I. Harbison (ed.) *Children of the Troubles, Children in Northern Ireland*, Belfast: Stranmills College.

Office for the Coordination of Humanitarian Affairs (OCHA) (2007) The Closure of the Gaza Strip: the economic and humanitarian consequences. Available online at: http://www.ochaopt.org/documents/Gaza_Special_Focus_December (accessed February 2009).

Palestinian Center for Human Rights website: http://www.pchrgaza.org/intifada.htm

Punamäki, R. L. (1984) *Reactions of Palestinian and Israeli Children to War and Violence*, Arab Studies Institute.

—— (1987a) *Children under Conflict*, Tampere: Tampere Peace Research Institute Report No. 23.

—— (1987b) *Childhood under Conflict. The Attitudes and Emotional Life of Israeli and Palestinian Children*, Tampere: Tampere Peace Research Institute Research Report No. 32.

—— (1990) Relationships between political violence and psychological responses among Palestinian women, *Journal of Peace Research*, 27: 75–85.

Pynoos, R. S. and Eth, S. (1985) Children traumatized by witnessing acts of personal violence: homicide, rape, and suicide behaviour, in S. Eth and R. Pynoos (eds) *Posttraumatic stress disorder in children*, Washington, DC: American Psychiatric Press.

Qouta, S. and El Sarraj, E. (1992) Curfew and children's mental health, *Journal of Psychological Studies*, 4: 13–18.

Qouta, S., Punamäki, R. L. and El Sarraj, E. (1995) Relations between traumatic experiences, activity and cognitive and emotional responses among Palestinian children, *International Journal of Psychology*, 30: 289–304.

—— (1996) House demolition and mental health: the victims and witnesses, *Journal of Social Distress and Homeless*, 6: 203–11.

—— (2003) Prevalence and determinants of PTSD among Palestinian children exposed to military violence, *European Child & Adolescent Psychiatry*, 12: 265–72.

—— (2007) Predictors of psychological distress and positive resources among Palestinian adolescents: trauma, child, and mothering characteristics, *Child Abuse & Neglect*, 31 (7): 699–717.

—— (2008) Does war beget child aggression? Military violence, child age and aggressive behaviour in two Palestinian samples, *Aggressive Behaviour*, 34 (3): 231–44.

Rachman, S. (1978) *Fear and Courage*, San Francisco: Freeman.

Rayhid, J., Shaya, M. and Armenian, H. (1986) Child health in a city at war, in J. W. Bryce and H. K. Armenian (eds) *Wartime: The State of Children in Lebanon*, Beirut: American University of Beirut.

Saigh, P. A. (1991) The development of posttraumatic stress disorder following four different types of traumatization, *Behavior Research and Therapy*, 29: 213–16.

Shanan, J. (1989) Surviving the survivors: late personality development of Jewish Holocaust survivors, *International Journal of Mental Health*, 17: 42–71.

Thabet, A. A. M., Abed, Y. and Vostanis, P. (2002) Comorbidity of PTSD and depression among refugee children during war conflict, *Journal of Child Psychology and Psychiatry*, 45: 533–41.

Thabet, A. A. M. and Vostanis, P. (1998) Social adversities and anxiety disorders in the Gaza Strip, *Archives of Disorders of Children*, 78: 439–42.

UN (2005) Protection of children affected by armed conflict, *Report of the Special Representative of the Secretary-General for Children and Armed Conflict*, 7 September, New York: Office of the Special Representative of the Secretary-General for Children and Armed Conflict. Available online at: http://daccessdds.un.org/doc/UNDOC/GEN/N05/483/03/PDF/N0548303.pdf?OpenElement (accessed 23 September 2009).

5.2 Childhood in the context of HIV/AIDS

The death of childhood

Gabriella Torstensson

Actively seeking the perception and experiences of children in these circumstances is the key to supporting their resilience and agency.

(UNICEF 2007: 5)

The human immunodeficiency virus (HIV), which is primarily but not exclusively transmitted through unprotected sex, and the advanced form of the disease, acquired immune deficiency syndrome (AIDS) were first detected in the early 1980s. Since then infection rates have soared and it is estimated that 39.5 million people are infected worldwide. HIV/AIDS now constitutes a global pandemic that is affecting individuals' and families' health, well-being, and financial and material sustainability and which is placing stress on key national and regional economies and social systems. However, global quantitative prevalence studies (that measure prevalence primarily by calculating the percentage of HIV positive women in antenatal clinics), have drawn the conclusion that the pandemic has now stagnated as new infection rates mirror death rates. This chapter argues that conclusions such as these often overshadow the enormous qualitative impact that the pandemic is having on children and the notion of childhood within the context of a growing AIDS pandemic.

This chapter focuses on the effect of HIV/AIDS on children's lives in Southern Africa, the pandemic's epicentre, and is based on several studies in the region. It places particular emphasis on the situation in Botswana, Zimbabwe and South Africa. A number of key contentions are presented, including:

- HIV/AIDS does not only affect orphans and vulnerable children (OVC), but affects all children's lives and well-being to various degrees.
- In the absence of a cure for AIDS, the only vaccine against AIDS lies in large-scale behaviour change.
- Actively seeking the perceptions, experiences, views and solutions of children is thus central to improving the effects of the pandemic and turning the trend around.
- The appropriateness of drawing on primarily Western views of childhood as outcomes of the mitigation process.

In essence, this chapter questions some of the conventional ways of exploring and measuring the impact of AIDS upon nations and children's lives and suggests that in order to find culturally sensitive solutions to the pandemic, we must actively begin to regard children as important protagonists in the fight against AIDS and seek to empower them to become agents of change. The analysis is structured around themes emerging from a study exploring children's perceptions of the impact of AIDS on their personal, family, community and school lives. This is followed by a discussion of the capabilities required in order for children to take an active role in alleviating the effects of the pandemic.

The HIV/AIDS pandemic in figures

Since the discovery of HIV/AIDS in the early 1980s, infection rates have escalated and by 2006 it was estimated that 39.5 million people worldwide were infected, with 4.5 million new infections alone in that year (UNAIDS/WHO 2006). Sub-Saharan Africa is hardest hit and hosts approximately 67 per cent of the world HIV infected population (UNAIDS 2008). The pandemic's epicentre is in Southern Africa, where 34 per cent of all people living with HIV/AIDS reside (UNAIDS/WHO 2006), with an infection rate of 33.4 per cent in Botswana (Seipone 2006), 30.2 per cent in South Africa (Department of Health South Africa 2006), 24 per cent in Zimbabwe (UNAIDS 2005) and 10–25 per cent in Zambia (Ministry of Health Zambia 2005). As a result of the pandemic, life expectancy has dropped in Southern Africa from above 60 to well below 40 (UNAIDS 2008). While it is argued that the pandemic has stagnated, as the new infection rates now mirror death rates (UNAIDS/WHO 2006), in the age group of many primary-school age children's parents (typically aged 25–35) infection rates continue to escalate (Seipone 2006), leaving many children bereaved as orphans (13.2 million between 1992–2001). By 2005, Sub-Saharan Africa had 12 million orphans and it is estimated that these figures will rise substantially over the next couple of years, with an orphan ratio of 20 per cent of children in Zambia and Botswana (UNAIDS 2008) and 24 per cent in Zimbabwe (UNAIDS 2008). Already in the late 1990s, Zambia had more than 130,000 child-headed families and 860,000 South African children had become teacher-less (Coombe 2001).

As global quantitative monitoring reports celebrate the perceived stagnation and the decline of new infections rates in adults in some nations, new data from Uganda, which had been portrayed as an example of how to curb the pandemic, indicate that infection rates are on the rise again in the 25–35 age group due to risky behaviour (UNAIDS/WHO 2006; UNAIDS 2008). Moreover, while it is important to take stock of the progress of the fight against AIDS, and as horrific as these figures are, to a large degree they mask the extent that the pandemic affects the lives of children.

Children's perceptions of the impact of HIV/AIDS

In a recent study exploring children's perception of the impact of HIV/AIDS on their own lives, their family, the community and their school life, primary-school age children in Botswana portrayed AIDS as a 'powerful killer disease that can't be stopped' (Pupil no. 25), one that 'does not choose its victims' (Pupil no. 24), as it 'kills mother, father, sister and brother' (Pupil no. 21) (Torstensson 2007: 122). An overwhelming number of children's pictures showed both young and old bedridden or with lesions and highlighted rib cages, as well as coffins, with the remaining family members grieving by the graveside, and many young children fending for themselves or being cared for by relatives. While only little more than half of the children had known or had seen people suffering from AIDS within their family, neighbourhood and the community, the majority of children described high levels of fear of contracting the virus or being orphaned. Girls described their fears of becoming infected through rape, being pressured into having sex against their will, having to engage in unsafe sex in order get money, being unable to negotiate safe sex or becoming infected by an unfaithful boyfriend or husband. Whereas some boys shared some of these thoughts, they also feared that they may become infected through fighting, or through the inability to negotiate safe sex as a result of alcohol intoxication. A few children also described a strong fear of becoming infected during their daily caring for younger siblings or parents who were HIV positive.

The majority of children had very good knowledge of AIDS, its symptoms and modes of transmission and prevention. However, in analysing children's statements, some demonstrated poor knowledge, such as believing that infection could occur through kissing, hugging, coughing and sharing baths, utensils and razors and this was associated with more frequent and stronger fears. For instance, a few children described how they were scared every time they saw their parents embrace, while some children were scared when parents displayed symptoms emanating from common colds, stomach bugs and fever. The fear that their parents should become HIV positive and die was strong and frequent in many children, regardless of their closeness of experience with AIDS. However, children in the urban areas described more horrific stories of what happened to children who became orphans and people who got AIDS. Their anxieties were exaggerated by frequent TV advertisements, TV and radio programmes featuring AIDS scenarios, and a lack of first-hand experience of what happened to orphans, as many were relocated to relatives in the villages or had had to fend for themselves. Children also described how more individualistic values in the urban areas meant that they had less trust in the community's ability and willingness to respect and care for them should they become orphans. Children's pictures also portrayed how children would help and care for each other, teach others about HIV/AIDS, and show compassion for those who were ill or affected. HIV/AIDS did not only feature strongly in their daily lives, but also in their perception of the future. All but a handful of students' visions of the future featured AIDS. While the mass media and an overwhelming majority of studies and government reports indicate that AIDS is primarily impacting on OVC, Torstensson (2007) concluded that in the context of AIDS, all children's socio-emotional lives, their behaviour, learning and attainment in school, as well as their perception of their own capacity to influence and take an active role in their own future and that of the nation, were affected to various degrees in countries and communities with high HIV/AIDS prevalence.

Living with AIDS in the family

A review of quantitative national and global AIDS prevalence reports would have us believe that the effect of AIDS on children's lives starts when they become orphans. This is partially due to the difficulties of measuring and monitoring the general well-being of all children, hence prevalence reports have had to rely on orphan statistics in order to measure the impact on children. However, a growing number of qualitative studies have found that the effect on children's psychosocial well-being begins when the child suspects that their parents may have AIDS. As a result of the stigma that surrounds HIV/AIDS, many of these children are suffering in silence. Fearing they will be blamed for their parents' illness, excluded from society or separated from their parents, many keep the illness to themselves. Both children and teachers noted how the worry and fear of having sick family members at home affected children's ability to spend time learning, socializing and playing, and building friendships. As the parental illness worsened, the child's decisions, time and opportunity to learn became increasingly dictated by the needs of the parents.

Many children whose parents were ill withdrew, became listless, anxious and quiet, and lost hope in the future. Many struggled to concentrate in school and complete their assignments (Torstensson 2007; Foster 2002). They increasingly felt powerless as the sickness pattern became so severe that the children could no longer predict what would happen from one day to the next. While grieving is often associated with loss, both Torstensson (2007) and Guest (2001) found that children showed signs of grieving when the parents were so ill that they could no longer show their love or provide guidance.

In addition to the psychosocial effect of having ill family members at home, acting as carers for their ill parents and younger siblings also meant an increased workload and a depleted family economy. Guest (2001) found that for many children in Zambia and Zimbabwe who had ill parents at home, schooling was no longer an option. While girls often had to leave school to care for the ill parent and for younger siblings, boys had to leave school to supplement the family income. However, in Botswana, where primary education is free and children receive free school meals, Bennell (2005) found the attendance of OVC was higher than in neighbouring countries, even though this became more random towards the later stages of the parents' illness.

Orphanhood

The concept of orphanhood is relatively new in many cultures in Sub-Saharan Africa, as traditionally children were brought up in extended family households on the father's side. When a parent died the child continued to be brought up collectively by the adults within the household. However, with the increasing migration to the cities in search for work and the breakdown of family structures, including less frequent contact with the extended family, children are now more likely to be brought up in more fluid family constellations, being cared for, for example, by an aunt or uncle, or grandparents while parents are working away in the cities. This phenomenon was more prominent in countries such as Botswana and South Africa, compared to Malawi and Uganda (Bennell 2005). Moreover, a review of studies of orphans indicates the definition of an orphan differs between studies and between nations. An orphan in the traditional Western sense is a child who has lost both parents. In many African cultures, however, orphanhood is connected to destitution (living below the poverty line), alienation, rootlessness, and the loss of social anchoring, support networks and connections with the extended family. Orphanhood within this context implies that that the extended family have failed in their traditional responsibility (Henderson 2006). Consequently, many orphans are never registered for the fear of bringing shame upon the family. Nor are they able to receive support and entitlement to free schooling from the government or other aid organizations. Nevertheless, the number of registered orphans has risen significantly in many areas of Southern Africa as can be seen from Table 5.2.1.

With the changing family constellations, traditional definitions of orphanhood, and the growing number of orphans in many countries, the incorporation of children into the extended family once a parent has died is more problematic than previously experienced. A review of studies exploring orphanhood in Southern Africa shows that factors such as family constellations, cultural values, economy, and the nauture of the new family influenced children's ability to feel settled.

For instance, in a study in a mining town in Zimbabwe, Matshalaga (2004) found that children cared for by grandparents felt happy, more loved and developed a stronger and rooted sense of identity than those cared for by aunts and uncles (see case study below)

Table 5.2.1 Number of registered orphans in Sub-Saharan Africa

	Registered orphans in 2001	*Registered orphans in 2007*
Botswana	57,000	95,000
Lesotho	37,000	110,000
Malawi	240,000	560,000
South Africa	400,000	1,400,000
Swaziland	19,000	56,000
Zambia	369,000	600,000
Zimbabwe	720,000	1,000,000

Source: UNAIDS (2008).

even though in the latter situation the children were financially and educationally better off and the children often had fewer family responsibilities.

Case study: Memory

Memory was 12 years old and lived with nine other cousins aged 3–13 and her grandmother Mai in a rural village in Zimbabwe. Mai was in her late 70s and had been blind for two years. The grandmother had cared for the orphans for the previous seven years since the death of her son. The household, which had no food reserves and was very poor, survived on the goodwill of a neighbour and her three daughters who were married. Memory and the other children sometimes had to go and look for food in the neighbouring homesteads. Although she was in her last year of primary school and there was an older boy in the household, Memory managed the housework and played the mother role for the rest of the children. After school she had to prepare the food for the other children, sweep the floor, clean the kitchen utensils and pots, do the chores, fetch water and firewood and supervise both the younger children and the other children doing their chores. She would often come home from school carrying her schoolbooks and fireworks on her head. During parent–teacher meetings, Mai would send a neighbour as a representative (Matshalaga 2004).

Similarly, children in Botswana described their grandparents as their insurance for future well-being, should their parents pass away (Torstensson 2007).

Case study: When friends are orphaned

A Year 5 pupil's account of what happened to two of her friends in urban Botswana when their mother passed away.

'The father told them that they could not live with him. The aunt started to look after them. The aunt was not kind to them, she told me. The aunt started to treat them like they were not her nephews and nieces. The grandmother took them when she saw that the aunt was not looking after them well. The grandmother was looking after six other children.'

Once the children were settled with their grandmother, the girl noted how her friends started to become happier again. However, she explained that she was not happier, because she wanted them to be able to live with their mother (Torstensson 2007: 150).

While Meintjes (2004) suggested that many orphans are not worse off than children from destitute families whose parents have to live and work away, respondents in Botswana contested this interpretation, as suggested by this head teacher's statement:

> 'Children who live with an aunt or uncle know that their mother might come on the holiday or the weekend. They know that they are there and that they care. But when the parents are dead, they surrender. They feel that they will never see their parents again.'
>
> (Torstensson 2007:149)

However, both Henderson (2006) and Torstensson (2007) found that children from single-parent households or from already fluid family situations more often continued to struggle to find stability and anchoring after the death of the parents, as can be seen in the case study below.

Case study: Happy Mbhele

Happy Mbhele, 13 years old, lived with her mother and little sister opposite her father's homestead in a rural area in South Africa. Happy's parents were unmarried and Happy seldom saw her father, who lived with his new family in Johannesburg. During the later stages of her mother's illness, when she suffered from constant diarrhoea, open blisters and sharp pains all over her body, fever and inability to maintain food, Happy was her main carer. She would have to wake up early in the morning to prepare hot water for her mother's bath and cook breakfast for her sister before she got ready for school, which sometimes started at six in the morning. Henderson (2006) noted how the girl was very thin and wore old threadbare clothes. Happy suggested that she had learnt to endure and be brave from her mother, who had been a hard worker, selling chickens and thatch grass to survive. After the mother's death Happy and her sister's living conditions were unstable. There was no direct incorporation of the children into the father's family, as the parents were never married, but their kinship with a new family was dependent on Happy's resourcefulness and continual search for a stable solution. The mother's relatives had not enquired about the children. Initially they went to live with her paternal uncle's wife, who was a widow with six children. At another point in time, they lived with her paternal grandmother, who was a traditional healer and rarely at home. As the children had hardly any food or even a candle to light at night when she was absent, they returned to the homestead of their paternal uncle's wife. The two girls also sought to find their father in Johannesburg, but were sent back without provision for their journey. Against the father's wishes, they returned to their paternal uncle's wife and stayed with her until they were old enough to live on their own. With her the children were able to continue schooling, even though they were unable to pay for school fees and supplies (Henderson 2006).

In the case of Botswana, head teachers and teachers noted that although there was a difference in the way that children settled and recovered within the new family – between children living with uncles and aunts or grandparents and those coming from nuclear families or single-parent households – the majority of children were well cared for and gradually began to return to their normal selves after approximately eight months. Only a handful of students continued to feel displaced and the majority of those had lost both parents and their siblings to AIDS (Torstensson 2007). As seen from all the case studies in this chapter, the closeness of siblings is an important factor in supporting children to deal with their grief, keep hope, muster up resilience to keep going, and overcome their difficulties. The need for sibling support is also reflected in the growing phenomena of child-headed families in Southern Africa, as can be seen in the case study below.

Case study: Honest and Janet

Honest, who is 12 years old, and Janet, who is eight, had lived together with their mother on the commercial farm in Zimbabwe where their mother had worked temporarily. They had no contact with their father and knew nothing of their mother's family background and were therefore not able to trace any of their relatives when their mother passed away. Instead they lived off handouts from the commercial farm community. The Farm Orphan Support Trust (FOST) secured funds so that the children could continue schooling and buy school-related equipment. Initially, the children were withdrawn, uncommunicative and sometimes aggressive, and their school attendance was poor. They were very protective of each other and it was hard to separate them into different classrooms. Their biggest fear was that they would be separated. As a result of FOST's work with the school in the form of training about AIDS orphans' needs and counselling skills, the children had a chance to deal with their grief and become more open (Walker 2002).

Activity 5.2.1: Vulnerability and resilience

- Can you explain how the children in the case above are both vulnerable and resilient?
- Reflect on what capabilities children would need to develop and what factors would contribute towards empowerment and the development of resilience.

At a first glance, the presence of child-headed families, that is families in which a child younger than 15 years of age shoulders the complete responsibility for younger siblings, may imply a breakdown in family ties. However, in studying families in Zimbabwe, Foster, *et al.* (1997) and Walker (2002) found that the factors that contributed to the establishment of child-headed families were numerous, ranging from: the rapid increase of parental death; reluctance of relatives to foster orphans for financial reasons and the lowering of family living standards; lack of contact with extended families; the presence of older siblings who have been the main carer during the parents' extended illness; fear of being separated from siblings; the dying parents' wish that the children should stay together; and fear of losing the family land, house and inheritance.

A review of research and case studies of orphans and their recovery suggests that there is a strong need for children to be closely connected with their siblings, to feel anchored within the community, and to feel like they are treated, loved and encouraged to take equal responsibility like other children in their new family. Henderson (2006) also found that children who had the opportunity to care for the parents before their death had developed greater resilience and ability to cope. Moreover, the ability to continue schooling provided not only a sense of hope for the future (Torstensson 2007; Henderson 2006; Walker 2002), but also an opportunity to be treated like all other children and have sense of normality (Torstensson 2007).

Schooling

With the exception of Botswana, where schooling is free, for many OVC in Southern Africa schooling is no longer an option. This is as a result of depleted family income, increased workload and relocation to households far away from school. Although the attendance of orphans in most countries is lower than non-orphans, figures indicate that in many countries that are worst hit by the pandemic governmental and non-governmental efforts and aid are slowly having an effect on orphans' ability to remain in education. Between 2003 and 2007, the school attendance of orphans increased by 2 per cent in Tanzania, almost 1 per cent in Swaziland, Zambia and Lesotho and more than 3 per cent in Mozambique, while in Zimbabwe and Gabon there was a decline in attendance (UNAIDS 2008). A recent study in Zimbabwe showed a direct correlation between the increase of AIDS within the country and an overall decline in academic grades. In Botswana, Torstensson (2007) found that not only were orphans and vulnerable children's educational attainments reduced by approximately two grades during the parental pre- and post-death period as a result of their own personal trauma, but the impact of AIDS on teachers' health and psychosocial well-being (which in turn caused high levels of teacher absenteeism) led to a decline in effective teaching and preparation. Consequently, all children who were taught in the same grade level as the sick teacher experienced a considerable loss of learning, as without the availability of a substitute teacher, classes were doubled when a teacher was absent. This effect was more severe in small two-form entry schools. This effect was more severe in small two-form entry schools as without the availability of a substitute teacher classes were doubled when a teacher was sick. The increases in class size from approximately 30:1 to 60–70:1 in Botswana and to over 80:1 in Zambia meant that teachers had to forgo effective interactive teaching methods, discussions and group work for less effective whole-class lecturing and copy work. Moreover, subjects that did not match these kinds of methods were taught less frequently or not at all during these sessions. Hence children experienced a decline in both breadth and depth of learning (Torstensson 2007). Although the cumulative loss of learning for OVC taught in the same grade level as a sick teacher was more severe, these findings suggest that all children's learning and attainments in areas with high HIV/AIDS prevalence are affected because of AIDS' impact on both the teachers' and pupils' ability to focus and be effective, as suggested by this teacher's statement:

> 'Many children are not happy. They are always thinking of death. They feel lost. They have seen it on television. They have heard from people talking. They are thinking that they will be dead in the future. They don't see a future for themselves. They are worried. They are thinking that they may have it too. Many are confused.'
>
> (Torstensson 2007: 223)

Although for many children remaining in schools is perceived as a ticket of hope, the effect of AIDS on their lives means that other children have given up hope for a better future. This in turn impedes their ability to be effective learners (Torstensson 2007; Walker 2002).

Children's perceptions of the future

A review of literature on the role of vision of the future indicates that a positive vision of the future is perceived as a strong motivational factor for behaviour change and empowerment (Laszlo 1989) and for the development of intrinsic self-esteem and motivation (Deci and Ryan 1995), acting as an anxiety buffer when faced with fear or mortality (Greenberg, et al. 1995). It provides direction and standards to judge development against and thus serves as a 'beacon in the fog' (Maurer 1996: 54). Consequently, a positive vision of the future may be perceived as an important attribute in the fight against AIDS, where the only vaccine is large-scale behaviour change. While Torstensson (2007) found that a negative vision of the future was clearly linked to disempowerment, the findings did not support a link between a positive vision of the future and greater empowerment. Rather, the study of the perception of the future of primary-school children in Botswana and their role in protecting themselves and taking an active part in turning the trend around indicated that factors such as cultural values and beliefs, closeness and the ability to contribute to the family and the community and to make links between the past, the present and the future played a greater part in translating knowledge of AIDS into healthy behaviour and a willingness and perceived ability to contribute towards mitigating the impact.

AIDS featured strongly in all but a handful of pupils' visions of the future, regardless of their level of experience of AIDS in the family, neighbourhood and the community, or the type of vision the children held. Their beliefs about the future, which ranged from 'Botswana will be a beautiful country, with big city and houses with electricity' to 'Botswana will be finished because of this killer disease' (Torstensson 2007: 157), can be divided into four categories, namely positive (31 per cent), wishful (16 per cent), dual (16 per cent) and negative (36 per cent) visions of the future. Children's positive visions of the future, which were predominately dependent on the eradication and the discovery of a cure for HIV/AIDS, focused on the material well-being and health of their families, community and country, as well as the development of the environment, social cohesion and human virtues. Believing in a positive vision, two groups of pupils either wished for a better future or explained that there could be two possible scenarios dependent on the behaviour change of people, the discovery of a cure, an increase in the numbers of nurses and doctors, and their own current behaviour and work in the future. The largest group of pupils (36 per cent) described an almost apocalyptic view of the future, where HIV/AIDS had destroyed families and communities, leaving children to fend for themselves. Some children thought that those left behind would struggle, have lots of problems and be scared most of the time, as suggested by this Year 6 pupil's account:

> 'By 2014 many people will be infected and others will die of this disease. Children will be left alone, but they too will die of this disease and of hunger. They will get food from the dustbins. They will run to have children. Their children will die because there will be no one to remind them. They will grow fatherless and motherless because their parents will be dead.'

> (Torstensson 2007: 3)

Others thought that even the children would be dead, and that the country would return to the state before people inhabited the land. Although this group of children had the greatest knowledge of AIDS symptoms, transmission and prevention, they had the least number of strategies to protect themselves and only a few children in this group thought that their actions would protect them against AIDS or help turn the trend around. The orphan respondents were divided equally between the positive and negative groups. While this may initially suggest that there is no link between orphanhood and a negative vision of the future, a closer analysis of the positive vision of orphans indicated that although some had settled well into their new families and felt genuinely hopeful about the future, others had not made a link between what had happened to their parents and their knowledge of HIV/AIDS. They had been told that their parents had died through witchcraft or by other disease, and that the illnesses that they saw in the communities were not caused by AIDS but rather linked to the anger of spirits. These findings were substantiated by an orphan worker who noted how orphans who had not made the link between AIDS and their parents' death struggled to see the importance of learning about AIDS, prevention strategies and capabilities to help turn the trend around. Orphans who had made this link showed greater willingness and empowerment to take an active role in their own future and their own health. Children in the two smaller groups who recognized the cause and effect of different types of behaviour and scenarios, described proportionally more strategies in which they could protect themselves as well as take an active role in turning the trend around. Many of these children had not only explored the different factors that increased the risk of infection but also described that it was vital that they developed skills, personal characteristics and virtues, as well as gain good grades in school, so that they could become nurses, doctors, teachers, community workers and leaders and share their knowledge with the people in the community. Hence, these findings support Nunn's (2006) argument that empowerment and change of behaviour is dependent on a thorough understanding of the past and the present, coupled with a realistic positive vision in the future for both ourselves and the world around us. Moreover, cultural values, the concepts and practice of equality, and connections with the community have also been found to be important factors in translating knowledge of AIDS into healthy behaviour (BIDPA 2003; Torstensson 2007).

Children as vulnerable victims or capable agents of change

A review of the data surrounding AIDS' impact on children, as seen from both children's and adults' perspectives, indicates that not only are all children within the context of AIDS more affected than the predominant quantitative studies would have us believe, all children are very vulnerable and to a large degree victims of circumstances beyond their control. However, there is a concern that with labels such as 'orphans' and 'vulnerable' children are objectified and easily become targets for AIDS-related stigma (Skinner, *et al.* 2004) and perceived as coming from families who have failed in their traditional responsibilities of caring for their offspring (Henderson 2006). Within the traditional definitions of orphanhood and vulnerability, such labelling can lead to greater feelings of exclusion, loss of connectiveness and anchoring within the community which can strip children of their rights and opportunities to play an active part in the development of the family and community. On the other hand, without such labels, children may lose out on valuable support and opportunities to continue schooling and become victims of abuse and neglect (Skinner, *et al.* 2004). Nevertheless, children in the Henderson (2006) study chose to reject the term 'orphan', rather seeing themselves as 'leaders of the future'. With such a term they perceived that both their agency and their role and status within society were maintained and raised. Torstensson (2007) found that close connections within the community were important in order for children to feel safe and to maintain a sense of trust in the future, and also highlighted the need for an opportunity to play an active part in helping those who were ill, teach about AIDS, and to be active in reducing AIDS-related stigma. This involvement helped to reduce their fears and contributed to the development of the children's confidence in their ability to protect themselves and to turn the trend around. Hence rather than seeing children in the 'centre', as a separate group around which the family and the community revolve as advocated in many Western societies, it may be more appropriate to regard children as being 'at the heart' of the family and the community. With such a notion, children are not only perceived as being at the centre of the life-giving organ of the family unit, but are also seen as competent from an early age and capable of playing a vital part in the 'pump stations' of the body of the family unit and the community. As noted by one head teacher and supported by a number of children in all studies, being perceived and treated like all other children in the family and being at the heart of the family, expected to take an active role in the family and contribute to their own and others' well-being, was important for successful incorporation into the new family and the speedy recovery after the death of a parent (Torstensson 2007).

Many children described great fears, anxieties and hopelessness and felt disempowered. Many felt a need to have somebody to talk to, opportunities to share their fears and anxieties and receive guidance. Many also showed courage and strength to question traditional norms that disallowed them to talk about AIDS and sex. They actively and openly discussed and guided both adults and the young about safe sex and relationships. Children in the studies and the case studies showed great compassion, strength, perseverance in adversity to care for those who were ill or were suffering, and insightfulness about the need for human character and moral development in order to help turn the horrific AIDS pandemic around. These are attributes which are not often associated with the terms 'vulnerable' and 'victims' in the general sense. Hence, basing mitigation strategies and support programmes on the notion of children being 'vulnerable' and not capable of participating in the process may in fact lead to disempowerment. While it is paramount to understand children's needs from both children's and adults' perspectives, within the context of AIDS it is also important to recognize and draw on children's views and understanding and to harvest their agency, as suggested by UNICEF (2007) in order to develop effective support strategies.

Many intervention programmes have primarily focused on short-term measurable goals such as condom distribution, the delivery of basic HIV/AIDS knowledge or school vouchers. However, when large-scale changes in behaviour and cultural practice are required, the solution lies in long-term strategies that touch the roots of the problem rather than simply seeking to address the symptoms of AIDS. Drawing on the views of children in the Bostwana study, children would need to develop qualities and virtues such as courage, patience, detachment, obedience to parents and skills in caring for others – in looking after orphans and people who were sick – without getting infected themselves. They would need to be able to set long-term goals, make decisions and develop the ability to forgo their immediate wants for long-term goals. Moreover, they described how they would need to be able to choose right from wrong and avoid getting into the wrong kind of company and have the ability to express and stand up for their own rights and wants and respect those of others, in order to avoid being pressured into risky situations. Children also describe the importance of having a good education so that they could become nurses and doctors and help find a cure for AIDS, as well as earning a living so that they could share and care for others and develop the nation. Moreover, they would also need to develop an understanding of gender equality and positive gender identities and the ability to analyse cultural values and norms, recognizing which lead to prosperity for all. And lastly, from the findings from children's perceptions of the future, children would need to be able to analyse and link the past, the present and the future.

As education is often perceived as the window of hope for the future, schools, in co-operation with children and communities, would need to provide opportunities for children to develop these capabilities. Without a cure for HIV/AIDS, their own behaviour and large-scale behaviour change within communities form the only vaccine the children have against HIV/AIDS.

Conclusion

This chapter has shown that although quantitative reports of the HIV/AIDS pandemic suggest that the pandemic has stagnated, as the number of new infections now mirrors the death rates, and the infection rates in some age groups have dropped, the continual reliance of primarily quantitative impact studies and HIV/AIDS prevalence indicators fails to adequately monitor and measure the pandemic's extent on children and their childhood. This chapter has questioned the accuracy and the usefulness of such conclusions when the orphan ratios continue to rise in all parts of the world and the extent of the pandemic does not only impact on OVC but stretches beyond and affects all children's lives, their well-being, perception of the future and ability to succeed in school in areas with high HIV prevalence, both now and in the future. While the context of AIDS has clearly made children more vulnerable, this chapter questions the usefulness of labelling children as vulnerable in the traditional sense. Rather, by drawing to a large degree on children's perspectives of the impact of AIDS on their lives and their community, this chapter shows not only that children play an important role in helping us to understand the impact of the pandemic but that channelling their knowledge, understanding, strength, passion, perceptions and perseverance, as well as strengthening their resilience and agency, is the key to mitigating the impact of HIV/AIDS and turning the trend around.

Activity 5.2.2: The 'vulnerable' label

- How can being labelled vulnerable lead to disempowerment?
- Consider how the plight of vulnerable children in the context of AIDS may compare to 'young carers' in Britain.

Student reflection

- How might our perceptions of childhood influence the way we treat children with serious illnesses such as HIV/AIDS and the extent to which we involve them in the decision-making process concerning the treatment of their illness and other aspects of their situation?

Key points

- In 2006 it was estimated that 39.5 million people were infected with AIDS worldwide, the majority being in Sub-Saharan Africa.
- This figure does not measure the impact upon children and childhood – by 2005 Sub-Saharan Africa had 12 million orphans.
- HIV/AIDS does not only affect orphans and vulnerable children (OVC), it affects all children's lives and well-being.
- Having AIDS in the family affects children in many ways, including the fear of being orphaned and worries about having to care for the family and being blamed for their parents' illness, in addition to affecting everyday life and learning.
- The closeness of siblings is a strong factor in helping children to deal with the various issues facing the family.
- Most children's perceptions of the future feature AIDS as a core aspect, ranging from it being a raging and destructive disease, to a cure being found and the well-being of their families being maintained.
- In the absence of a cure for AIDS, the only vaccine against AIDS lies in large-scale behaviour change and children can be key elements in the fight against AIDS by being empowered to become agents of change.
- Actively seeking the perception, experiences, views and solutions of children are thus central to improving the effects of the pandemic and turning the trend around.

Recommended reading

Cornia, G. A. (2002) *AIDS, Public Policy and Child Well-being*, Florence: UNICEF.
Dow, U. (2000) *Far and Beyond*, Gaborone: Longman.
Fox, J. (2002) *Nkosis' Story*, Johannesburg: The Life Story Project/Spearhead.
Guest, E. (2001) *Children of AIDS*, Pietermaritzburg: Pluto Press.

References

Abt Associates (2002) *Impact of HIV/Aids on the Botswana Education Sector: Summary*, Gaborone: Abt Associates and Botswana Ministry of Education.
Bennell, P. (2005) 'The impact of AIDS pandemic on the schooling of orphans and other directly affected children in Sub-Saharan Africa', *Journal of Development Studies*, 41 (3): 467–88.
BIDPA (2003) *Knowledge, Attitudes and Practices of Teacher and Students on HIV and AIDS: Baseline Study Report*, Gaborone: Botswana Institute for Development Policy Analysis.
Coombe, C. (2001) *HIV/AIDS and Trauma among Learners*, Pretoria: National Union of Educators.
Deci, E. L. and Ryan, R. (1995) 'Human autonomy – the basis for true self esteem', in M. H. Kerris (ed.) *Efficacy, Agency and Self-esteem*, New York: Plenum Press.
Department of Health South Africa (2006) *National HIV and Syphilis Antenatal Prevalence Survey, South Africa 2005*, Pretoria: Department of Health South Africa.
Foster, G. (2002) 'Beyond education and food: psychosocial well-being of orphans in Africa', *ACTA Paediatrica*, 91 (5): 502–4.
Foster, G., Makufa, C., Drew, R. and Kralovec, E. (1997) 'Factors leading to the establishment of child-headed households: the case of Zimbabwe', *Health Transition Review*, 2 (7): 155–68.
Greenberg, J., Pyszczynski, T. and Solomon, S. (1995) 'Towards a dual motive depth psychology of self and social behaviour', in M. H. Kerris (ed.) *Efficacy, Agency and Self-esteem*, New York: Plenum Press.
Guest, E. (2001) *Children of AIDS – Africa's Orphan Crisis*, Scottsville: University of Natal Press.

Henderson, P. (2006) 'South African AIDS orphans – examining assumptions around vulnerability from the perspectives of rural children and youth', *Childhood*, 13 (3): 303–27.

Laszlo, I. (1989) *The Inner Limits of Mankind*, London: One World.

Matshalaga, N. (2004) *Grandmothers and Orphan Care in Zimbabwe*, Harare: SAfAIDS.

Maurer, R. (1996) *Beyond the Walls of Resistance*, Austin: Bard Press.

Meintjes, H. (2004) 'Spinning the epidemic: the making of mythology of orphanhood in the context of AIDS', paper presented at the 'Life and Death in the Time of AIDS: the Southern African Experience' symposium, Wits University, October.

Ministry of Health Botswana (2005) *2005 Botswana Second Generation HIV/AIDS Surveillance Technical Report*, Gaborone: Ministry of Health Botswana.

Ministry of Health Zambia (2005) *Zambia Antenatal Sentinel Surveillance Report 1994–2004*, Lusaka: Ministry of Health Zambia.

Nunn, K. (2006) 'Neurofuturity: a theory change', *Journal of Clinical Psychology and Psychiatry*, 11 (2): 183–90.

Seipone, K. M. D. (2006) *Trends of HIV Prevalence in Botswana: Department of HIV/Aids Prevention and Care*, Gaborone: Ministry of Health Botswana.

Skinner, D., Tsheko, N., Mtero-Munyati, S., Segwabe, M., Chibatamoto, P., Mfecane, S., Nkomo, N., Tlou, S. and Chitiyo, G. (2004) *Defining Orphan and Vulnerable Children*, Cape Town: Human Science Research Council.

Torstensson, G. (2007) 'Managing the impact of HIV/Aids in Botswana's education system: redefining effective teaching and learning in the context of AIDS', unpublished doctoral thesis, Leicester University.

UNAIDS (2005) *Evidence for HIV Decline in Zimbabwe: A Comprehensive Review of Epidemiological Data, November*, Geneva: UNAIDS.

—— (2008) *Report on the Global AIDS Pandemic*, Geneva: UNAIDS.

UNAIDS/WHO (2006) *AIDS Epidemic Update*, Geneva: UNAIDS, December.

UNICEF (2007) *The State of the World's Children 2007 Executive Summary*, New York: UNICEF.

Walker, L. (2002) *'We Will Bury Ourselves' – A Study of Child-headed Households on Commercial Farms in Zimbabwe*, Harare: Farm Orphan Support Trust of Zimbabwe.

Wyze, D. (ed.) (2004) *Childhood Studies: An Introduction*, Oxford: Blackwell.

5.3 Moving for a better life

To stay or to go

Samantha Punch

Child migration is a relatively new area in academic and policy debates although in practice this is not a new phenomenon. At the beginning of the twenty-first century there was very limited literature available, but over the past five years or so this has begun to change, partly as a result of research programmes such as those being carried out by the Development and Research Centre on Migration, Globalization and Poverty, and the UNICEF Innocenti Research Centre.

Most of the literature on migration has focused on adults and rarely have migrant children's own perspectives been heard. Consequently, inadequate assumptions have been made about child migrants' lives. For example, it has been assumed that children migrate because they are forced to: coerced by their parents for economic reasons or trafficked by others to be prostitutes or slaves. They are often portrayed as passive victims of exploitation, lacking agency and not having an active role in the decision-making or migration process (Hashim 2006).

Farrow (2007) argues that this is because children have tended to be viewed as migrating only as dependants rather than as independent migrants. As a result of this focus on more harmful situations, children's migration experiences have usually been assumed to be negative: they suffer poor working conditions; receive very low (or even no) pay; and have no access to education. Such generalizations have disguised the reality of many migrant children's lives.

Recently some studies have explored ordinary children's everyday lives in the majority[1] world in a variety of contexts, such as rural Uganda (Bell 2007), rural Bolivia (Punch 2003) and suburban South Africa (Benwell 2008). Children being forced to migrate and working in exploitative conditions may be the case for some young migrants, but for many it is not. For example, Riisøen, *et al.* point out that in their studies in Burkina Faso, Ghana and Mali, 'trafficking still represents a relatively limited practice when considering the extensive relocation of children taking place in the region' (2004: 54).

This chapter explores the complexity and diversity of children's migration motives and experiences, first in relation to work and second in relation to education. It begins by discussing the multiple reasons for the migration of children, and subsequently their positive and negative experiences. It draws mainly on the emerging literature in this field as well as the author's own research with young migrants who leave southern rural Bolivia to work in a nearby town and in neighbouring Argentina (Punch 2002; 2007a).[2] Most of the child migrants discussed in this chapter are older children, in the 13–18 age range (also referred to here as 'young people'), as there is a paucity of literature which considers the much smaller group of migrants who are under 13 years of age.

Activity 5.3.1: Migration of the young

The focus of this chapter is on children and young people who migrate for work and education.

- List the reasons why you think young people may migrate for work and education.
- List the benefits you think they may gain and the negative experiences you think they may have to cope with.

Types of migration

There are many different types of migration which both adults and children engage in. Lynch (2005) identifies a range of movements between rural and urban areas

> ... including step-wise migration (village – town – city), circulatory migration (village – city – village), cyclical migration (associated with seasonal variation in labour demand), multi-locational households (where households have members in town and country) and chain migration (where migrants follow their predecessors, are assisted by them in establishing an urban base).
>
> (96)

Migration is often a dynamic process involving a variety of movements between households in different areas. Many young immigrants move back and forth between their home community and migration destinations. Furthermore, many migrants do not just settle in one location but may move on seasonally or yearly depending on available opportunities or difficulties that arise. Thus, young migrants may move through a variety of jobs and move on to different places. This may be seasonal according to where the work is, or it may be opportunistic and based on who they meet. New friends may introduce them to new opportunities or they may decide to move on somewhere different together. Hence independent child migration can be mobile and flexible, resulting in uncertain pathways and fragmented youth transitions. Migrants can live precarious lives being quite dependent on changes in global and local economies. Consequently, they have to be flexible in order to adapt to changing circumstances both in the wider environment and in their private lives (moving through the life course, having children, parents getting older and needing more support etc.). As Ansell says in relation to her research in Southern Africa, 'The labour migration complex is not static, but constantly evolving' (2000: 155).

Migration is a widespread coping strategy for economically poor households as by diversifying their livelihood options they reduce their risks and vulnerability (Yaqub 2007). Many households in the majority world depend on migrant remittances for survival (Francis 2000). Children routinely contribute to the economic maintenance of their households from an early age in a range of different ways (Punch 2001). Thus, migration of children and young people is another way that they actively participate in their own and their household's livelihoods. In the minority world this is not a common experience and work is not a key component of the way childhood is socially constructed. However, globally more children live in the majority world so the experience of child migration is fairly significant and is central to many rural livelihoods, even though reliable statistics are difficult to find to illustrate this. Furthermore, as work is central to many majority world childhoods (Punch 2003), the fact that children seek migrant work opportunities is unlikely to be culturally unacceptable or perceived as inappropriate by the children themselves or by their parents. Hence we need to move away from minority world assumptions that independent child migration is a necessarily exploitative or damaging experience for children.

Decision-making process

Like all aspects of migration, the decision-making process around whether children should migrate or not is extremely diverse and complex. Parents and children may influence the decision to varying degrees. Siblings can also have an important role in this process (Punch 2002), and in particular birth order can be crucial in determining when a young person migrates (Punch 2001). Sometimes both children and parents may be quite ambivalent about whether the young person should stay or go. It is often not a clear-cut decision that is made easily. Return migrants inspiring others to leave should not be underestimated as an influential factor in the decision-making process (Castle and Diarra 2003). For example, Riisøen, *et al.* suggest that 'The aspect of curiosity and peer pressure may tempt children from well off and stable households to leave home in search of adventure' (2004: 52).

The important point is that children are not just passive pawns but often actively seek migration opportunities themselves. For example, in Bourdillon's study (2007) of child domestic workers in Zimbabwe, two-thirds of the children said they chose to seek employment and some older children took it for granted that they should be working (72 per cent of the sample were aged 15–18, and 28 per cent were under 15). In Camacho's research (1999) with child domestic workers in the Philippines, 80 per cent of the children said it was their personal decision to work.

Therefore, sometimes parents are instigators or actively encourage their children's migration, sometimes they resist it and try to postpone it and sometimes they may be actively against it and children leave without their consent (Iversen 2006). For example, Punch (2001) found that in Bolivia some parents were keen for their children to migrate later when they were a few years older, partly because they needed more help on the land with the animals or agriculture. Some children had to wait a year or two until their siblings were old enough to take on their household jobs and often a compromise was reached about when they could leave. Thus, as Hashim argues: 'children do make strategic life choices and negotiate with adults to do so' (2006: 26). Ultimately the decision to migrate is made within a range of opportunities and constraints, and can be for individual reasons or family reasons, but often it is a combination of both.

Migrating for work: reasons

Recent research has indicated that there are multiple reasons why children migrate for work. One of the key underlying factors is poverty but the motives are often not purely economic as there are many other social and cultural reasons why children seek migrant work. At the macro level there are a range of crises which may lead to children's migration, such as political conflict (Boyden and de Berry 2004), economic crises, HIV/AIDS (Ansell and van Blerk 2004) and environmental disasters (Lynch 2005). Global economic restructuring and uneven development has led to increased levels of migration as young people leave impoverished rural areas in search of employment and better lifestyles

(Bryceson 2004). For some communities out-migration is a relatively new phenomenon (Carpena-Mendez 2007) but for others there may already be a long history of migration (Ansell 2000). For example, favourable exchange rates in particular can encourage international migration particularly across borders such as from Mexico to the US (Hellman 2008) or from Bolivia to Argentina (Bastia 2005).

Development, or the lack of it, also shapes migration flows. For example, in parts of Eastern and Southern Africa urban labour markets are overcrowded and new migrants can be unable to find work, which has resulted in some migrants moving back to rural areas (Francis 2000). Swanson (2007) describes how a new road built in 1992 has opened up migrant work opportunities for women and children in Calhuasí, Ecuador. Thus processes of development can impact on levels of both out-migration and return migration.

For children and young people in rural subsistence communities migration may be necessary if they have no access to land, which is often the case unless their parents lend them land or they have inherited land. Their work opportunities may be very limited, particularly during the dry season if there is a lack of irrigation systems. Lack of available land can become increasingly problematic as family plots are divided up for the next generation resulting in insufficient land for each child to inherit (Swanson 2007).

At the micro level of the household, some children end up migrating as a result of domestic violence or abuse (Iversen 2002), or personal crisis and gender-based discrimination (Bastia 2005). At the community level, Whitehead and Hashim (2005: 25) point out that in areas where there are high rates of adult migration there can also be high rates of child migration. This is particularly the case in communities that have a 'culture of migration', where young people may feel left out if they have never migrated (Bey 2003). If there is a long history of migration from that area, then migration may be the norm and may be encouraged by return migrants and by parents who see it as an opportunity for their children. Camacho (1999) explains that:

> The family does not only transmit work-related values, it also transmits migration-related values to its members. ... The cultural context of the community likewise may socialize children towards work-related migration.
>
> (68)

Hashim (2006) argues that there are two key benefits for migrants from areas with a long history of migration. First, there are wider social networks as extended families become dispersed and second there is a greater knowledge of alternative labour markets. Both of these mean that the likelihood of getting work is increased and the decision to migrate may be easier compared with those who live in areas that do not have a culture of migration. Thus the availability of social networks influences a child's decision to migrate. If they know they are likely to get work in their migrant destination, can travel with others and stay with others on arrival then this is likely to increase their likelihood of deciding to leave. Camacho (1999) indicates that having family-based contacts at the place of destination could facilitate children's decision to seek employment as domestic workers in the Philippines.

For many young people migration is strongly linked to their stage in the life course as it becomes important for their transition from childhood to adulthood (Carpena-Mendez 2007). Migration is like a 'rite of passage' which many young people feel a need to experience on their pathway to a more economically and socially independent lifestyle. Both parents and children in Thorsen's study spoke about 'being awake' (2005: 11) after having lived in a town or city, referring to becoming mature, responsible and more autonomous. Children in Hashim's research cited that 'their interest in new life-experiences' (2006: 26) was a reason for leaving and girls migrated to 'have their eyes opened' (Hashim 2005: 33). Curiosity to 'see what it's like' and not be left behind (Bey 2003) should not be underestimated as an important motive for encouraging children to migrate.

Similarly, linked to the notion of a 'rite of passage' and youth transitions, becoming economically independent is a key reason why children seek migrant work in order to be able to consume more widely and access global goods, as well as save for the future (Punch 2007a). Whitehead and Hashim (2005: 28) argued that a central motivation for migration is children's 'need or desire for income'. Thorsen (2005) found that children in her study in Burkina Faso used their income to buy clothes and possibly a bicycle if they could earn enough.

Children's motives for migration often include meeting their individual needs and their obligations of contributing to the household. This balancing act is referred to elsewhere as 'negotiated interdependence' (Punch 2002), a term

> ... which reflects how young people in the majority world are constrained by various structures and cultural expectations of family responsibilities yet also have the ability to act within and between such constraints, balancing household and individual needs.
>
> (Punch 2002: 132)

Similarly, Hashim (2006: 26) found that children in her study in Ghana saw themselves 'as economic agents with a responsibility to contribute to their households and their individual livelihoods' and Camacho argues that 'family and personal goals are interwoven' (2007: 64) for the children in her study in the Philippines.

Migration also enables young people to actively participate in constructing new opportunities for their future (Jeffrey and McDowell 2004). For example, it opens up possibilities of them staying at the migrant destination, moving on to another place of migrant work or returning back home to their community of origin. Thus migration can lead to broadening their future opportunities and opening up of new choices, albeit limited ones. Finally, another reason why children may migrate in search of work is because there may be a lack of education opportunities at home which may lead to them seek work instead.

Migrating for work: experiences

Recent research with independent child migrants has highlighted the variety and complexity of children's migratory experiences. For some children their experience is more negative, and for others it is more positive overall, but often there is a mixture of both advantages and disadvantages for the same migrant. Perhaps a useful question to ask is: What are the criteria for 'successful' migration? For example, is it the ability to save money and accumulate resources, or is it to do with emotional happiness, perhaps meeting a partner? Is it individual success or being in a position to contribute more to the household back home, or is it learning new skills? Furthermore, is return migration perceived to be a good or bad thing? Some people hate the arduousness of migrant work, in particular the long hours and the poor conditions, and they may rather have less money but be in their home setting instead of being an unwelcome outsider in a hostile environment (Punch

2002). Other migrants can bear those hardships because of the opportunity to earn higher levels of income (Hashim 2006: 16). Hence, it is important to seek the young migrants' own views regarding their positive and negative experiences of migration.

Positive benefits of migrating that have emerged in the recent literature are closely linked to the reasons why children decide to migrate, as discussed previously. Migration can be a learning experience, a 'rite of passage' where children become more socially and economically independent. The majority receive material benefits, often a higher income than they could earn in their home community, which gives them access to more consumer goods and enables them to send remittances home and contribute more to their family. Migration can offer an opportunity to learn new skills, such as different agricultural techniques or even new domestic skills. Even though this is often a reason for new migrants to be paid less in their first job or for an initial period, the new skills can be beneficial. Other social benefits include meeting new people, seeing new places and experiencing new things (Castle and Diarra 2003).

The availability of social networks at the migrant destination can also enhance the likelihood of children having a more positive migrant experience. However, even when things go badly, children often develop coping strategies and build up resilience, and this can lead to them gaining self-confidence from their ability to cope (Boyden, *et al.* 1998). Furthermore, working at a migrant destination is not always tougher than experiences of working back home so it can seem relatively more positive in comparison to what they are used to (Johnson, *et al.* 1995). By seeking migrant work children are opening up a wider range of future options, albeit limited ones, as they may then be able to decide whether to stay, move on, or return. Sometimes they may also enable their younger siblings to benefit as their remittances can be used to pay for their siblings' studies (Bourdillon 2007). Furthermore, migration may enable children to create a new identity and this may be either positive or negative.

Ansell and van Blerk (2007) found that in their study of children in Lesotho and Malawi the migrant identity was stigmatizing, but for other young migrants it can enhance their social status. For example, for many children having a migrant identity when back home in their rural community in Bolivia was very positive and was perceived to be an important part of their youth identity (Punch 2007a). In Mexico, Carpena-Mendez (2007) found that migrant children could blur the boundaries between urban and rural identity. This thus emphasizes how a particular experience for one set of young migrants can be experienced very differently by other migrants. Furthermore, as other personal factors intervene, children's migration experiences should only be considered as positive or negative (or both) on an individual basis.

Negative experiences can be particularly marked at the beginning of the migrant journey, as the process of leaving home for the first time can be emotionally difficult and overwhelming (Ansell and van Blerk 2007). Many young migrants talk about loneliness and homesickness especially at first, but to varying degrees. While learning new skills can be a positive aspect of migration, it can also be problematic especially while having to adapt to a new environment. The working conditions can be arduous for some migrants, such as very long hours, low pay, having to work in the heat or with flies. Living conditions can also be difficult to endure, such as a lack of space and comfort, cramped sleeping arrangements or insufficient food. Having limited social networks in the migrant destination can make it much harder for migrants to cope. Some migrants may suffer physical, verbal, or sexual abuse from their employers or others at their place of work, and many describe different levels of stigma or discrimination attached to their migrant position.

The extent to which migration is a positive or negative experience can depend on a wide range of factors, with most migrants moving back and forth between positive and negative experiences in different contexts, with different people, and at different times of the migration process. As Yaqub says, 'Children's vulnerability is not an absolute state. There are degrees of vulnerability, depending on the situation of the child' (2007: 6). Thus, migrant children experience shifting vulnerabilities in different contexts or aspects of their lives, and their highs and lows move back and forth on a continuum according to different factors. Therefore, the process of migration can be both empowering and disempowering and young migrants may feel both empowered and disempowered in different ways at the same time (Punch 2007b).

In a sense, migration can be empowering as it enhances young people's economic and consumer power, enabling them to buy material goods and clothes which they would not otherwise be able to afford. This, along with the wider horizons they have experienced, can increase their status among their peers. Also, by contributing economically to their household, they earn more decision-making power and more control over their use of time and space when back home. They may feel relatively powerless in the migration destination, but have increased power and status back home. As Camacho (2007: 65) states, overall children felt positive about the migration experience, as they felt that the benefits to themselves and their families compensated for the hardships and difficulties they experienced.

Intergenerational relationships and intra-generational relationships

It is important for research to consider how inter- and intra-generational relations are renegotiated over time, and that they may involve both co-operation and conflict. Independent child migrants by definition leave their community without their parents (Whitehead and Hashim 2005). Their parents may have their own personal histories of migration or they might not have ever migrated before and it may lead to tensions or conflicts of interest. When the children return home either for a short visit or for longer periods there can be a clash of values between the generations, between old and new ideas (Taracena 2003). For example, Bryceson (2002) gives examples of young people who return after migrating and question authority at both the household and community level. In rural Bolivia, some of the older generation disapproved of the younger return migrants partying and drinking alcohol because in their eyes they were 'wasting' their migrant earnings (Punch 2007a).

Intergenerational relationships can also be mutually supportive and Hashim (2006) discusses the role of the 'inter-generational contract' in relation to children's migration. Thorsen (2005) describes parents giving children advice on how they should behave away from home, and some helped out by paying the transport for their child. In the available literature on children's independent migration, most of the discussion of household relationships focuses on children's relations with their parents rather than their intra-generational relationships with siblings. Siblings can also play an important role in the migration process both during decision-making and at the destination, particularly if their parents have never migrated before. Punch (2007b) found that siblings were often an extremely crucial source of support: sharing their migrant experiences, travelling together, or helping them seek work.

Youth transitions

Given that it is a relatively new focus of migration literature, independent child migration is under-theorized. The concept of 'youth transitions' may be a useful framework to understand some children's processes of migration. Youth transitions do not just refer to transitions from school to work, or from unpaid work to paid work, but also include other kinds of transitions, such as leaving home, forming a new household, developing new relationships, getting married, and having children. Many of these impact upon the decision to migrate as well as shape the experience of migration. For example, once children leave home, migration means they have to find new living arrangements and sometimes this leads to them forming their own household. This may involve acquiring housing and/or access to land for the present and/or for the future. If opportunities for building or acquiring their own house arise, this is likely to influence their decision on whether to stay or return. Young people may meet their partners or future spouses during their process of migration. Depending on when and where they meet, they may have to decide how to combine their migrant experiences and destinations (they may be working in different places) and previous families (sender communities). If they have children and start a new family of their own, this leads to further decisions regarding whether to migrate as a family or whether the wife and children will stay behind, and if so, in whose household? The nature of different youth transitions may thus shape the type of migration which young people undertake.

Migration for education: reasons

For many young people living in rural areas in the majority world, if they wish to continue to secondary education they have to migrate as only primary education is available nearby (Ansell 2004). Schools in rural areas can be under-resourced and the teaching quality can be poor which may lead young people to migrate to better schools (Bey 2003). In some parts of the majority world, young people are under pressure to continue schooling because an educated identity is linked to increased status (Jeffrey, *et al.* 2004). Many children end up combining work and education by migrating to work in order to pay for school themselves because their parents are not able to support them (Camacho 1999). Hashim (2005) gives examples of children migrating to work for certain periods of time and then going back home to continue their schooling. The availability of 'fostering' situations can also provide children with an opportunity to continue their education (Hashim 2005). For example, some children in Bolivia would go and live with relatives or friends in town, helping out with a range of domestic chores in return for free board and lodging while they attended school.

The key motivation underlying all of the above reasons to migrate for education is to improve their future employment prospects. However, many children end up rejecting migration for education and choose work instead for a range of reasons. For example, the structural constraints of education in rural areas can lead to young people rejecting further schooling as an option for improving their future livelihoods. This includes constraints such as limited resources, lack of available teaching materials, inadequate infrastructure and poor quality of teaching and low wages for teachers (Punch 2004) which all lead to a poor perception of schooling. Some children do not continue with their education because they feel under pressure to start earning an income and have access to cash (Aitken, *et al.* 2006). For other children, the more tangible benefits received by migrating for work can mean that migration for education seems less attractive (Levinson 1996). Some have a realistic view that in their socio-economic context pursing education is unlikely to lead to a better livelihood; it can be a large financial sacrifice, but with a very uncertain outcome (Punch 2004). Thus, it can be rational for children to give up schooling where labour markets are limited and structured, as they may not be able to obtain formal employment afterwards. As with the decision to migrate in order to work, the decision to migrate for education can also be influenced by parents and/or siblings to varying degrees.

Migration for education: experiences

Similar to children's migrant work experiences, it is likely that their migrant education experiences are both positive and negative and that these change over time and in relation to different aspects of their daily migrant lives. However, there tends to be an assumption that continuing education is a good thing and there is not much research which discusses the negatives of pursuing an education as a migrant (except Jeffrey, *et al.* 2004 who discuss the difficulties of becoming educated and then not being able to get work). In fact, besides Hashim (2005) there seems to be limited research that explores children's views of what it is like to migrate for education. Camacho briefly discusses child domestic workers' experiences of combining their work with education, attributing 'their academic difficulties to the heavy workload leaving them little time to study, or being too tired to pay attention in class' (1999: 62). Camacho (2007) has also argued that if children are working in order to pay for their own schooling, then household resources can be used to send their siblings to school. However, on the whole, we know little about what happens to children who decide to continue their education rather than migrate for work, or who combine migrant work and education, and the extent to which they have positive or negative experiences.

Activity 5.3.2: Attitudes to education

- Can you explain the differences in attitudes to education described in this chapter with the attitudes of many children within the UK?
- What factors can you identify that influence a child's attitude to education?

Punch (2004) in a follow-up study in Bolivia, recorded the negative experiences of a 22-year-old who previously left a rural area and migrated for education to an urban area. The woman stated that as a girl she felt that she would never fit in in the city. She did not have the same economic resources as the other children to buy clothes, uniform and books. She spoke differently to the others and she found that the demands of the urban school and the standards of schooling there were different than those she had experienced in the countryside. Eventually she left the school and returned to her home.

Influential factors

Children's reasons for migrating and their subsequent experiences can be shaped by a range of factors including the social, cultural and economic contexts, gender, age and household composition. The cultural context shapes whether children migrate or not, depending on whether there is a tradition of migration and on the cultural meanings attached to 'childhood' and 'migrant work'. The social context, in terms of available social networks and parents' attitudes (supportive or not), and the economic context, in terms of available work and education opportunities and constraints, also both influence the likelihood of whether children migrate or not.

Children's experience of work can be affected by gender, as the type of work can be strongly gendered: 'they often enter the same labour market as adult migrants from the same area' (Whitehead and Hashim 2005: 30). Hashim (2005: 32) found that girls are less embedded in the social, cultural and economic relations of the community in Ghana and so are more able to migrate than boys, being seen as temporary household members. A key reason for girls migrating can be to save to buy things for marriage and to learn a skill to have their own possibility for income generation. The evolving capacities of the child impact upon their migration experiences. For example, Hashim (2006) found that younger children (7–13 years) had less active involvement in the decision to migrate, whereas older children (13–18 years) were more likely to choose to migrate, often having to negotiate with parents in order to be able to.

Many of the examples given in this chapter tend to be in relation to older children, 13 to 18 years old. There is much less research available with the younger age group, partly because the majority of independent child migrants are 13 or above. Riisøen, *et al.* (2004) state that as a child gets older the reasons for migrating change. The stage in the life course is an important factor which influences children's decision to migrate or not. Further research is needed, in particular with children under 13 years of age in order to explore the differences between the younger and older age groups.

Whitehead and Hashim point out that 'Many of [migration's] positive and negative effects do not arise from the fact of migration itself, but depend on what triggers movement, what kinds of circumstances migrants move to and, of course, the distance moved and the length of stay away' (2005: 45). It is worth bearing in mind that this can be as much about migration for work as for education. Therefore, other factors that may affect the quality of children's migratory experience include the reason for migrating, the type of work/school, the migrant location, the climatic conditions, the working/studying/living conditions, the relationship with employer/teacher, availability and accessibility of social networks, the length of migration and opportunities for visits back home.

Conclusion: child migrants' constrained choices

The evidence seems to suggest that many child migrants are able to cope and build up resilience, but we do need to remember that often their migration experience is a coping strategy to enable them to get by within the structural constraints that they face. They can assert their agency to a certain extent but it is within structural limits. Children may have positive migrant experiences but this is relative to the wider negatives that surround their lives. In other words, they have limited options or alternatives. Many are migrating to work as domestic maids or on agricultural plantations or in other low paid, low skilled, low status jobs. They come from areas that lack opportunities and development, so, as Hashim points out, 'These children are exercising agency to choose the least worst option' (2006: 28). Thus, research with independent child migrants should consider both children's agency and structural constraints:

We need to understand how different migratory contexts alter the balance of children's agency and opportunities on the one hand, and risks and vulnerabilities on the other.

(Yaqub 2007: 3)

As Camacho (2007) says, we should be trying to move away from polarizing children's experiences:

> … acknowledging the complexities and subjectivities in children's migration experiences calls for an approach that rejects the conventional contrast between children as passive pawns and vulnerable preys or as active and autonomous agents in the migration process.

(65)

Therefore, we need to think more in terms of a continuum of experiences and try to strike a balance between exploring the range of positives and negatives that exist at both the sender and destination communities. We should strive to consider the different arenas of migrant children's everyday lives, rather than just focusing on their work or education experiences, and combine different perspectives: both adults' views (parents, employers, teachers) and children's opinions (siblings, friends, peers). It is also important to explore the impact of both intergenerational and intra-generational relationships on the migration process. Finally, when exploring both children's agency and the structural constraints they work within, it is appropriate to consider how these change over time as they move through the life course.

Student reflection

Having read this chapter, consider your thoughts on child migration.

- Do you consider child migrants to be victims or agents in making decisions about their own lives and futures?

Key points

- Child migration, though not a new phenomenon, is a relatively new area of research and academic study.
- What research there is on child migration tends to see children as victims of trafficking for prostitution or slavery or as forced to migrate due to warfare or diseases such as AIDS. The child is seldom seen as a decision-maker in the migration process.
- In reality, many children migrate of their own volition for work and/or education. They are frequently supported by their parents, siblings and wider community and they may be from a culture in which migration is the norm and, indeed, is often seen as 'a rite of passage'.
- Children migrate for work for macro reasons, e.g. political conflict, poverty, development or lack of it, and for micro reasons, e.g. domestic violence or abuse, gender discrimination.
- Young people may migrate to continue secondary education or for better schools, resources, teaching. Frequently child migrants combine work and education, though many eventually give up education for the economic benefits to themselves and their families of work.

- The experiences of young migrants range along a continuum of positive and negative. Some negative experiences are homesickness, loneliness, poor working conditions, insufficient food and physical or sexual abuse.
- The benefits of migration can be: economic rewards for the migrant and their family, broadening of horizons, improved future prospects, educational achievements, gaining in respect and status with peers and family.
- It is important to remember that while many young people do choose to migrate their choices are often limited and may constitute the best choice among other bad ones. Also, as children grow and mature their range of choices and their agency over their choices also changes.

Notes

1 The more recent terms 'minority world' and 'majority world' will be used in this chapter to refer to the developed and developing world respectively. These terms invite us to reflect on the unequal relations between the two world areas. The minority world consists of a smaller proportion of the world's population and land mass despite using the majority of the world's resources.

2 This included ethnographic research for the author's PhD on children's everyday lives in rural Bolivia conducted during July 1993 to July 1995, and July to December 1996, and a four-month follow-up study from April to July 2006. During the follow-up study (funded by the British Academy) 14 of the original 18 sample households were traced in order to explore what the children had done in the ten years since the original study. Only five of the school pupils aged 8–14 years in 1996 were still in the community in 2006. Over half had migrated to work in Argentina and others had migrated to the nearby town of Tarija. Girls tended to migrate to domestic work and boys to agricultural plantations in the north of Argentina. Only three were continuing with their secondary-school education in Tarija.

Recommended reading

Marfleet, P. (2006) *Refugees in a Global Era*, Basingstoke: Palgrave Macmillan.
Panelli, R., Punch, S. and Robson, E. (2007) (eds) *Global Perspectives on Rural Childhood and Youth: Young Rural Lives*, London: Routledge.
Watters, C. (2008) *Refugee Children: Towards the Next Horizon*, London: Routledge.
Yaqub, S. (2007) *Migrant Unaccompanied or Separated Children: Issues and Knowledge Gaps*, Florence: UNICEF Innocenti Research Centre.

References

Ansell, N. (2000) 'Sustainability: life chances and education in Southern Africa', in M. Redclift (ed.) *Sustainability: Life Chances and Livelihoods*, London: Routledge.
—— (2004) 'Secondary schooling and rural youth transitions in Lesotho and Zimbabwe', *Youth & Society*, 36 (2): 183–202.
Ansell, N. and van Blerk, L. (2004) 'Children's migration as a household/family strategy: coping with AIDS in Malawi and Lesotho', *Journal of Southern African Studies*, 30: 673–90.
—— (2007) 'Doing and belonging: toward a more-than-representational account of young migrant identities in Lesotho and Malawi', in R. Panelli, S. Punch and E. Robson (eds) *Global Perspectives on Rural Childhood and Youth: Young Rural Lives*, London: Routledge.
Aitken, S., López Estrada, S., Jennings, J. and Aguirre, L. M. (2006) 'Reproducing Life and Labor: global processes and working children in Tijuana, Mexico' *Childhood: A Global Journal of Child Research*, 13(3): 365–388.

Bastia, T. (2005) 'Child trafficking or teenage migration? Bolivian migrants in Argentina', *International Migration*, 43 (4): 57–80.

Bell, S. (2007) '"The child drums and the elder dances?" Girlfriends and boyfriends negotiating established power relations in rural Uganda', in R. Panelli, S. Punch and E. Robson (eds) *Global Perspectives on Rural Childhood and Youth: Young Rural Lives*, London: Routledge.

Benwell, M. (2008) 'Social geographies of childhood: outdoor spaces, mobility and "growing up" in post-apartheid suburban Cape Town, South Africa', unpublished PhD thesis, Royal Holloway and Bedford New College.

Bey, M. (2003) 'The Mexican child: from work with the family to paid employment', *Childhood*, 10 (3): 287–300.

Bourdillon, M. (2007) 'Child domestic workers in Zimbabwe: children's perspectives', in B. Hungerland, M. Liebel, B. Milne and A. Wihstutz (eds) *Working to be Someone: Child Focused Research and Practice with Working Children*, London: Jessica Kingsley.

Boyden, J. and de Berry, J. (eds) (2004) *Children and Youth on the Front Line: Ethnography, Armed Conflict and Displacement*, Oxford: Berghahn Books.

Boyden, J., Ling, B. and Myers, W. (1998) *What Works for Working Children*, Stockholm: Rädda Barnen and UNICEF.

Bryceson, D. (2002) 'The scramble in Africa: reorientating rural livelihoods', *World Development* 30 (5): 725–39.

—— (2004) 'Agrarian vista or vortex: African rural livelihood policies', *Review of African Political Economy*, 102: 617–29.

Camacho, A. Z. V. (1999) 'Family, child labour and migration: child domestic workers in metro manila', *Childhood*, 6: 57–73.

—— (2007) 'Understanding the migration experiences of child domestic workers: towards alternative perspectives on children and migration', paper presented at the 'Focus on Children in Migration' conference, 20–21 March, Warsaw, Poland.

Carpena-Mendez, F. (2007) '"Our lives are like a sock inside-out": children's work and youth identity in neoliberal rural Mexico', in R. Panelli, S. Punch and E. Robson (eds) *Global Perspectives on Rural Childhood and Youth: Young Rural Lives*, London: Routledge.

Castle, S. and Diarra, A. (2003) *The International Migration of Young Malians: Tradition, Necessity or Rite of Passage?*, London: London School of Hygiene and Tropical Medicine.

Farrow, C. (2007) 'A review of European research findings on children in migration', paper presented at the 'Focus on Children in Migration' conference, 20–21 March, Warsaw, Poland.

Francis, E. (2000) *Making a Living: Changing Livelihoods in Africa*, London: Routledge.

Hashim, I. (2005) *Exploring the Linkages between Children's Independent Migration and Education: Evidence from Ghana*, Working Paper T12, Development Research Centre on Migration, Globalization and Poverty, University of Sussex.

—— (2006) *The Positives and Negatives of Children's Independent Migration: Assessing the Evidence and the Debates*, Working Paper T16, Development Research Centre on Migration, Globalization and Poverty, University of Sussex.

Hellman, J. A. (2008) *The Rock and the Hard Place: The World of Mexican Migrants*, New York: The New Press.

Iversen, V. (2002) 'Autonomy in child labour migrants', *World Development*, 30 (5): 817–34.

—— (2006) *Segmentation, Network Multipliers and Spillovers: A Theory of Rural Urban Migration for a Traditional Economy*, Working Paper T9, Development Research Centre on Migration, Globalization and Poverty, University of Sussex.

Jeffrey, C. and McDowell, L. (2004) 'Youth in a comparative perspective: global change, local lives', *Youth & Society*, 36 (2): 131–42.

Jeffrey, C., Jeffery, R. and Jeffery, P. (2004) 'Degrees without freedom: assessing the social and economic impact of formal education on Dalit young men in North India', *Development and Change*, 35(5): 963–86.

Johnson, V., Hill, J. and Ivan-Smith, E. (1995) *Listening to Smaller Voices: Children in an Environment of Change*, Somerset: ACTIONAID.

Levinson, B. A. (1996) 'Social difference and schooled identity in a Mexican secundria', in B. A. Levinson, D. E. Foley and D. C. Holland (eds) *The Cultural Production of the Educated Person: Critical Ethnographies of Schooling and Local Practice*, Albany, NY: State University of New York Press.

Lynch, K. (2005) *Rural-urban Interaction in the Developing World*, London: Routledge.

Punch, S. (2001) 'Household division of labour: generation, gender, age, birth order and sibling composition', *Work, Employment & Society*, 15 (4):803–23.

—— (2002) 'Youth transitions and interdependent adult-child relations in rural Bolivia', *Journal of Rural Studies*, 18 (2): 123–33.

—— (2003) 'Childhoods in the majority world: miniature adults or tribal children?', *Sociology*, 37 (2): 277–95.

—— (2004) 'The impact of primary education on school-to-work transitions for young people in rural Bolivia', *Youth & Society*, 36 (2): 163–82.

—— (2007a) 'Negotiating migrant identities: young people in Bolivia and Argentina', *Children's Geographies*, 5 (1): 95–112.

—— (2007b) 'Generational power relations in rural Bolivia', in R. Panelli, S. Punch and E. Robson (eds) *Global Perspectives on Rural Childhood and Youth: Young Rural Lives*, London: Routledge.

Riisøen, K. H., Hatløy, A. and Bjerkan, L. (2004) *Travel to Uncertainty: A Study of Child Relocation in Burkina Faso, Ghana and Mali*, Norway: Fafo.

Swanson, K. (2007) '"Bad mothers" and "delinquent children": unravelling anti-begging rhetoric in the Ecuadorian Andes', *Gender, Place and Culture*, 14 (6): 703–20.

Taracena, E. (2003) 'A schooling model for working children in Mexico: the case of children of Indian origin working as agricultural workers during the harvest', *Childhood*, 10 (3): 301–18.

Thorsen, D. (2005) *Looking for Money while Building New Skills and Knowledge: Rural Children's Independent Migration in South-Eastern Burkina Faso*, Field Report, Development Research Centre on Migration, Globalization and Poverty, University of Sussex.

Whitehead, A. and Hashim, I. (2005) *Children and Migration: Background Paper for DFID Migration Team*, London: Department for International Development.

Wyn, J. and Dwyer, P. (1999) 'New directions in research on youth in transition', *Journal of Youth Studies*, 2 (1): 5–21.

Yaqub, S. (2007) *Migrant Unaccompanied or Separated Children: Issues and Knowledge Gap*, Florence: UNICEF Innocenti Research Centre.

Index

Entries in **bold** denote references to figures and tables.